21 THINGS
YOU NEED TO KNOW ABOUT
DIABETES

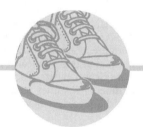

and
your
FEET

Neil M. Scheffler, DPM, FACFAS

American
Diabetes
Association.

Director, Book Publishing, Abe Ogden; *Managing Editor,* Greg Guthrie; *Acquisitions Editor,* Victor Van Beuren; *Editor,* Rebekah Renshaw; *Production Manager,* Melissa Sprott; *Composition,* ADA; *Cover Design,* Jody Billert; *Printer,* United Graphics, Inc.

Printed in the United States of America
3 5 7 9 10 8 6 4 2

The suggestions and information contained in this publication are generally consistent with the *Clinical Practice Recommendations* and other policies of the American Diabetes Association, but they do not represent the policy or position of the Association or any of its boards or committees. Reasonable steps have been taken to ensure the accuracy of the information presented. However, the American Diabetes Association cannot ensure the safety or efficacy of any product or service described in this publication. Individuals are advised to consult a physician or other appropriate health care professional before undertaking any diet or exercise program or taking any medication referred to in this publication. Professionals must use and apply their own professional judgment, experience, and training and should not rely solely on the information contained in this publication before prescribing any diet, exercise, or medication. The American Diabetes Association—its officers, directors, employees, volunteers, and members—assumes no responsibility or liability for personal or other injury, loss, or damage that may result from the suggestions or information in this publication.

♾ The paper in this publication meets the requirements of the ANSI Standard Z39.48-1992 (permanence of paper).

ADA titles may be purchased for business or promotional use or for special sales. To purchase more than 50 copies of this book at a discount, or for custom editions of this book with your logo, contact the American Diabetes Association at the address below, at booksales@diabetes.org, or by calling 703-299-2046.

American Diabetes Association
1701 North Beauregard Street
Alexandria, Virginia 22311

DOI: 10.2337/9781580404778

Library of Congress Cataloging-in-Publication Data

Scheffler, Neil M.
  21 things you need to know about diabetes and your feet / by Neil M. Scheffler, DPM, FACFAS.
    pages cm
  Includes bibliographical references and index.
  ISBN 978-1-58040-477-8 (alk. paper)
  1. Foot--Diseases--Popular works. 2. Diabetes--Complications--Popular works. 3. Foot--Care and hygiene--Popular works. I. American Diabetes Association. II. Title. III. Title: Twenty-one things you need to know about diabetes and your feet.
  RC951.S34 2012
  616.4'62--dc23

                          2012036748

"This book is dedicated to my wife, Eleanor,
who puts up with all the time I spend on my computer.

Thanks also to those podiatrists
who helped train me during my residency:
Drs. Irvin Donick, Larry Block, Steven Berlin and Lanny Rubin.
I can never thank you enough."

Table of Contents

Diabetes and Your Feet

Diabetes has become an epidemic in this country. This epidemic is costing hundreds of billions of dollars each year in direct and indirect costs while destroying the lives of those with this disease, as well as those of their friends and families. The personal costs to patients include financial as well as non-economic, emotional, social, and psychological burdens. The risk for death among people with diabetes is about twice that of people of similar age without diabetes.

According to data from the 2011 National Diabetes Fact Sheet, 25.8 million children and adults in the United States—8.3% of the population—have diabetes. 79 million people have prediabetes. 1.9 million new cases of diabetes were diagnosed in people aged 20 years and older in 2010, and there is no end in sight. Diabetes rates in adults ages 65 and up may surge in the next 20 years as the population of senior adults is expected to double to more than 71 million by 2030.

Lower extremity complications of diabetes account for more in-patient hospital days than any other complication of the disease. More than 60% of lower-limb amputations due to causes other than trauma occur annually in people with diabetes; this number is more than 65,000.

If you want to be active and independent all of your life—whether or not you have diabetes—you need to have healthy feet. Most people take their feet for granted, but people with diabetes do not have that luxury. You are challenged by complications of diabetes that can make it easier for you to develop a foot ulcer that may not heal. Nonhealing ulcers often lead to amputation, which will severely limit what you can do for yourself.

The good news is that by taking good care of your feet, you can often prevent diabetic foot complications. If you take care of your feet every day and get good medical care as soon as you suspect you might need it, you're much more likely to avoid getting the infections that make amputation necessary. According to the Center for Disease Control (CDC), "comprehensive foot care programs, i.e., those that include risk assessment, foot-care education, and preventive therapy, treatment of foot problems, and referral to specialists, can reduce amputation rates by 45% to 85%."

This book will help you protect your feet. You will learn about the major lower extremity complications of diabetes: vascular disease (circulation problems), diabetic neuropathy (nerve problems), and foot deformities (such as bunions and hammertoes). You will see how these can affect your feet, how to prevent them, or, if they do happen, what you can do about it. Reading this book is the first step in preventing amputations and keeping your feet happy and healthy. Let's get started!!

Diabetes Foot Care Team

Perhaps you have heard about the "team approach" to treating diabetes. You may be interested in putting together a team for your foot care. Who should be on this team? How often should you see them and what should you expect?

The most important member of the team is YOU. You need to practice good foot hygiene, wear your prescribed shoes and inserts, and in general take charge of your own foot health. You need to assemble your team and help them to help you.

A podiatrist is a foot and ankle specialist who you should see at least once a year. If you have foot problems, such as poor circulation, nerve problems, wounds, or deformities you will need more frequent visits. You can see a podiatrist for routine foot care if you are unable to reach or see your feet. Podiatrists are doctors of podiatric medicine (DPM) and, in most states, diagnose and treat conditions of the feet and ankles. They perform routine foot care, such as toenail trimming, callus removal, and treatment of ingrown toenails, and they perform foot surgery on bones and soft tissue, such as bunion or hammertoe surgery. If necessary, a podiatrist can operate on infected bones and do amputations (some orthopedists do foot surgery as well). Podiatrists study how your feet and legs work when you move and walk (biomechanics). Podiatrists can identify bone and joint deformities that put unusual pressure on the skin of your feet. They can design insoles or braces to help your feet work normally and order special footwear if you need it. Podiatrists are trained in the treatment of the diabetic foot, including the treatment of wounds and infections. Your podiatrist will do a thorough history and exam and should treat any current problems and advise you about preventing future foot issues. He/she should suggest changes in shoes and socks. You should call your podiatrist immediately if you see any changes in your feet.

Your podiatrist should work closely with your primary health care provider (PCP). In fact, you may already have had a PCP before you chose your podiatrist. Your PCP is an excellent person to ask for a referral to a podiatrist or any medical specialist. Your PCP is the go-to person for any medical problems you may have. Your PCP and podiatrist may suggest these other members of your team:

> Vascular surgeons specialize in surgery on blood vessels and can help restore circulation to your feet. If your feet are cold or you notice your feet looking red or blue you may have poor circulation and require the expertise of a vascular surgeon. Vascular surgeons often help heal wounds and prevent gangrene and amputations.

> A neurologist may join the team if you have neuropathy (numbness or pain due to abnormal nerve function). The neurologist may perform nerve testing and prescribe medications to decrease pain or numbness.

> A physiatrist (a physician specializing in rehabilitation medicine) and a physical or occupational therapist may be consulted if you need rehabilitation. Physiatrists may also test nerves and help treat neuropathy or chronic pain.

> A pedorthist is a professional who fits shoes and insoles for people with foot problems. Pedorthists do not diagnose or prescribe care; they should follow the advice of your podiatrist or primary care physicians. When you visit a pedorthist make sure you have your doctor's prescription or recommendation with you.

- A certified diabetes educator (CDE) can help teach you how to care for your feet.

- A nutritionist or registered dietician (RD) can help you with your diet plan to assist in your efforts to control your diabetes. Good control may help prevent complications such as peripheral neuropathy.

- An endocrinologist can help with your diabetes management. Good control of your diabetes may be able to prevent complications such as diabetic neuropathy.

Your family members who help you care for your feet at home are also part of your health care team. Family members or friends can be especially important if you cannot see your feet to examine them, or if you cannot reach your feet to clean or treat them.

Have a complete foot examination at least once a year. During this exam, your health care provider or podiatrist will look for any changes in shape (deformity) that alter the way you walk and bear weight on the foot. He or she will also check for loss of feeling by pressing a thin plastic wire that looks like a piece of fishing line, called a monofilament, against the soles of your feet or by holding a vibrating tuning fork against the base of your big toe. The provider will check your circulation and examine your skin, especially between your toes and under the metatarsal heads (the bones in the ball of your foot). If you can't examine your own feet or if you have foot problems or nerve damage, have your feet checked more often, probably at every visit to your health care provider.

The following are warning signs. You should have your feet checked immediately if you have any of these symptoms.

- pain, redness, swelling, or increased warmth

- a change in the size or shape of the foot or ankle

- pain in the legs at rest or while walking

- tingling or numbness in the feet

- open sores (with or without drainage), no matter how small

- nonhealing wounds

- ingrown toenails
- corns or calluses with skin discoloration
- unexplained high blood glucose levels

Diabetic Neuropathy

About 60% to 70% of people with diabetes have mild to severe forms of nervous system damage. The results of this damage can include impaired sensation or pain, muscle weakness in the feet or hands, slowed digestion of food in the stomach, carpal tunnel syndrome, erectile dysfunction, or other nerve problems. Almost 30% of people with diabetes over the age of 40 have impaired sensation in the feet (i.e., at least one area that lacks feeling). Severe forms of diabetic nerve disease are a major contributing cause of lower-extremity amputations.

Peripheral neuropathy is the name for damage to sensory, motor, and autonomic nerves. Motor and sensory nerves help you move and feel the world around you. In the feet, autonomic nerves control perspiration. Autonomic neuropathy may result in dry, cracked skin. "Peripheral" means at the edges or away from the center, or away from the brain and spinal cord. In this case, the feet are farthest from the center of the body. "Neuro" means nerves and "pathy" means "a disorder of." Because the longest nerves are usually affected first, symptoms such as tingling, burning, or numbness appear first in the feet and hands.

You can think of the nervous system like the electrical system in your house. The wires to the lights and appliances are the peripheral nerves, and the fuse box and the main electric cable are the central nervous system (the brain and spinal cord). When motor nerves are damaged, muscles in your foot can become weak and allow the shape of the foot to change. Toes can curl up, and the fat pad on the bottom of the foot can shift so that it no longer protects the skin on the bottom of the foot. Bones can get very close to the skin and can cause calluses. The sensory nerve damage prevents you from feeling pain, so a callus can become an ulcer without you being aware of it. Autonomic nerve problems can cause dryness of the skin.

While it is not yet known how diabetes causes nerve damage, it is likely that higher than normal blood glucose levels are part of the cause. Keeping your blood glucose levels close to normal can lower your chances of developing neuropathy. People with high blood glucose levels are more likely to have neuropathy, and the longer a person has diabetes, the more likely he or she is to experience this complication. Researchers are working to better understand the causes of neuropathy and to find treatments to avoid the damage that it causes.

If you have had diabetes for more than 10 years and you have not kept your blood glucose levels close to normal, you likely have some symptoms of nerve damage. It affects as many as 75% of all people with diabetes. Symptoms can range from muscle weakness, cramps, numbness, tingling, pins and needles, and burning sensations, to changes in bowel habits, bladder control, or sexual functioning. Your may also notice that your feet bother you more at night. Even unexplained episodes of fainting or vomiting can be attributed to nerve damage.

Although there is no one specific test that all doctors use to check for neuropathy, there are some that are widely accepted. Your doctor may touch your feet with a small, thin fiber called a monofilament. If you can't feel this light touch, you have lost sensation. Similarly, you should be able to feel the vibrations of a tuning fork on your feet. A nerve conduction study, which tests the speed of electrical transmission through the nerves, may also be used. A trained neurologist or physiatrist will be consulted to perform this test.

Three types of neuropathy are associated with diabetes: autonomic, sensory, and motor. In the feet, autonomic neuropathy affects perspiration and the dryness of the skin. Although this dryness can be a problem, it does not change the shape of the feet.

Sensory neuropathy affects how the feet feel. This type of neuropathy causes numbness, burning, tingling, and/or pain. If your feet are numb, you often will not feel pain, and you may walk on a foot that is being damaged. You may also step on a nail or piece of glass and not know it. A Charcot foot is a breakdown of the structure of the foot—multiple fractures and a destruction of the bony architecture. The arch area may become so deformed it looks convex rather than concave.

Motor neuropathy affects the way the muscles work. The muscles deteriorate and over time, patients with longstanding diabetes and motor neuropathy may lose as much as half of the muscle volume of their feet. When the muscles of the foot do not work properly, an imbalance occurs and toes are often pulled out of their normal position. These are called hammertoes. When the toes move upward, they also pull with them soft tissue structures like the fat pad on the ball of the foot. This increases pressure on the bottom of the foot, and calluses and ulcers often form. These deformities must be addressed.

The best treatment for neuropathy is to keep your blood glucose levels on target. Studies show that near-normal blood glucose levels can also help prevent nerve damage from getting worse. If you have painful neuropathy and start taking insulin or oral medications to lower your blood glucose, you may notice a short increase in pain until your body becomes accustomed to the lower blood glucose levels.

Medications such as antidepressants, anticonvulsants (seizure medicine), muscle relaxants, local anesthetics (such as a lidocaine patch), and anti-inflammatory drugs, as well as vitamins, evening primrose oil, and capsaicin creams made from hot peppers, have been used to treat neuropathy symptoms.

Capsaicin is a substance found in hot peppers. Capsaicin cream removes a chemical—substance P, from the nerve ends below your skin and may interrupt your feeling pain. Apply it lightly several (3 to 4) times a day. Wear gloves or wash your hands carefully after applying capsaicin—you do not want to get hot pepper cream in your eyes, your mouth, or any other sensitive area! When you first use capsaicin, you may have a stinging or burning sensation that should disappear in a few days to a few weeks. Don't give up just because it burns.

Do not use capsaicin if you are sensitive or allergic to hot peppers. Capsaicin cannot be used on damaged or irritated skin, wounds, or rashes. Don't put tight clothing or bandages over the cream. Use it 3 to 4 times a day for 3 to 4 weeks before deciding whether it is working. Since capsaicin comes in different strengths, discuss what strength to use with your health care provider.

Physical therapy treatments such as stretching exercises, massage, and electrical nerve stimulation have also been tried. Some doctors have reported success with surgery performed on affected nerves. Although studies of these therapies report some improvement in painful symptoms for some patients, there is no single treatment that works for everyone. It may be difficult to get complete relief. Discuss your symptoms with your provider and try the treatment you both think might work. If that treatment doesn't help, let your provider know so you can try another one.

Numbness in your feet is a very serious condition. Most people go to the doctor because their feet hurt, but may not realize if they've lost sensation. It is important to look at your feet and touch them every day. Keeping your blood glucose on target may help prevent the numbness from getting worse. See your podiatrist regularly. You may also need to have your shoes fitted properly by a pedorthist (certified shoe fitter) and find out whether you need special shoes to protect your feet. Check your shoes before each wearing for foreign objects, nails, or anything that may injure your foot. Be sure your socks are not wrinkled or twisted. You may want to switch to socks without a toe seam, because seams can put too much pressure on your toes.

If you find that the numbness is uncomfortable, discuss treatments for neuropathy with your health care provider. Whenever there is any injury to your feet or a change in shape or a change in the skin, see your foot care specialist right away. Do not wait until an infection develops!

A decrease in foot sweating can be a sign that diabetic nerve damage is occurring in the nerves that control sweating. This is called autonomic neuropathy. However, foot sweating also tends to decrease as we age, especially if we become less active. Wearing different shoes or socks can affect foot sweating, as well. You may have recently started wearing shoes that do not hold in moisture, so your feet are drier.

The problem with a decrease in foot sweating, whatever the cause, is that the foot skin tends to become very dry and prone to cracking. Cracks in the skin may become infected. It is a good idea to use a moisturizing cream or lotion on your feet (but not between the toes) if you have dry skin.

An unsteady gait can be related to diabetic nerve damage. When a person has loss of feeling in his or her feet, the positioning system of the body does not get normal responses about where the feet are being placed. This can cause the person to feel unsteady or to trip and stumble. An unsteady gait can be a sign of other problems, too—some of which can be quite serious. If you are having trouble with your balance or walking, talk with your provider about a consultation with a neurologist or physiatrist.

If your unsteadiness is due to nerve damage, it may be time to get a cane. It's better to be safe and use a walking aid than to risk a fall and a broken hip! Your provider or physical therapist can help you get the right length and give you tips on how to walk with a cane. A physical therapist can also teach you balance exercises and how to increase awareness of the position of your feet.

Sometimes diabetes-related muscle weakness can contribute to unsteadiness in walking. Your provider or physical therapist can show you muscle-strengthening exercises. Some people need a lightweight brace or ankle support to stabilize the ankles when muscle weakness is the problem.

Not all pain or numbness in your feet may be diabetes related. Some vitamin deficiencies, such as vitamin B12, can cause neuropathy. A neuroma (sometimes called Morton's neuroma) can manifest itself with tingling, burning, or pain in your two middle toes. At first this problem may only occur when you wear tight shoes, but the numbness and pain will eventually progress so you feel pain in any shoes. Compression of a nerve in this area, between the third and fourth toes, causes the nerve to thicken and creates these symptoms. People with and without diabetes may get neuromas. Treatment for this problem may include shoe inserts (orthotics), wider shoes, injections of cortisone, injections of alcohol to "kill" the nerve, or surgery to release pressure on the nerve or to remove the neuroma entirely.

Peripheral Vascular Disease

One of the most serious complications possible in people with diabetes is peripheral vascular disease (PVD) or peripheral arterial disease (PAD). PAD is commonly called "poor circulation" and refers to blockage in the blood supply, often to the feet. A buildup of plaque inside the arteries that carry blood to the feet causes them to thicken and harden. Plaque is a substance that lines artery walls and is made up of calcium, cholesterol, fat, and other substances found in the bloodstream. People without diabetes get this thickening and hardening of the arteries as well, but unfortunately these problems can happen sooner and can be more severe in people with diabetes. PAD is 20 times more common in people with diabetes than in the general population. Other things that put you at risk of developing PAD are smoking, poor nutrition, lack of exercise, high blood fat levels (including cholesterol), and high blood glucose levels. Gangrene, or the death of tissues, is the most serious stage of PAD.

You can help to avoid or limit PVD by stopping smoking and keeping your blood fats and blood glucose levels as close to normal as possible. See a registered dietitian (RD) for help with your meal plan and add more physical activity to your lifestyle.

Your primary care physician, your endocrinologist, and your podiatrist should check you for PAD at least once a year. He or she will ask about cramping in your legs when you walk and will examine your feet and legs and feel for pulses, located in the groin, behind the knee, at the ankle, and on top of the foot. You may need to have the blood pressure in your ankles, arms, legs, and toes checked. (The arteries in toes don't get stiff, so measuring blood pressure there may be more accurate.) A Doppler machine may be used; this test is painless. Some experts suggest that people with diabetes who are over the age of 50 should have a baseline Doppler exam (also called an ankle brachial [arm] index) to compare the blood pressure in their feet and arms. You may need a test to measure how much oxygen gets to the skin of your feet.

If you have an ulcer that won't heal, or areas of your foot that break down despite wearing properly fitted shoes, you may need special X-rays and scans. These tests take pictures of the blood flow from your thigh to your toes. For arteriogram X-rays, you get an intravenous injection of a special solution so that the blood vessels show up clearly on the X-ray. This solution is called "dye," although it really does not change the color of anything. People with poor circulation should consult with a vascular surgeon—a doctor who specializes in this type of problem. If you have questions, ask your provider and the people performing the tests to explain things to you.

The hallmark sign of poor circulation is pain or cramping in the calf or the thigh (usually the calf) that occurs when you walk a short distance. This pain is a sign that the muscles are not getting enough oxygen. If you slow or stop and rest for a few minutes, the oxygen supply usually catches up with the demand and you can walk a little farther before the pain reoccurs. The medical term for this condition is "intermittent claudication." Claudication is similar to angina in people with poor circulation to the heart, except it occurs in the leg muscles. With angina there is chest pain that is relieved by resting the heart.

Other signs of poor circulation are pain at rest, nonhealing ulcers, absent or weak pulses in the feet or legs, a decrease in blood pressure in the feet and legs, or a lack of hair growth on the lower legs. A blue or purplish color, especially when your feet are hanging down, is also a sign of circulation problems.

If you think you may have poor circulation, ask your provider to evaluate it. Poor circulation is caused by a blockage in the arteries supplying blood to the feet. The blockage may need to be removed or bypassed with vascular surgery. A simple treatment is to walk every day. This exercise can force the body to form new blood vessels and improve the circulation in your feet and legs. Having poor circulation in your feet also puts you at greater risk for heart disease.

Cold feet may be a sign of poor circulation; however, many things can cause cold feet, so it's not necessarily a circulation issue. If you think you have poor circulation, have your feet evaluated by your health care provider. The best thing to do for cold feet is to wear one or two pairs of thick socks or warm house slippers—but check to be sure that your shoes are not too tight. Try the thin silk socks that are worn under regular socks for added warmth. There are also special socks available that warm feet safely. Getting up and walking around or getting regular exercise helps keep your feet warmer.

Do not use heating pads or hot water bottles on your feet. Don't sit too close to a space heater, fireplace, or campfire. If you have any diabetic nerve damage, you cannot feel when your feet are too hot or are getting burned, and you could be badly injured. In addition to making your feet feel cold, nerve damage can affect blood flow and sweating in the feet. It's best to wear socks and get up and move around.

Smoking is clearly connected to developing cardiovascular (heart and blood vessel) disease. When you smoke, the combustion products of tobacco are absorbed into the bloodstream. These chemicals stimulate the release of other chemicals, which injure the blood vessels and encourage thickening and hardening of the arteries. Smoking also causes your blood vessels to constrict, or clamp down, limiting the amount of blood that can circulate. Because the constriction of the blood vessels by tobacco lasts for hours, smoking even as few as two cigarettes a day can affect your circulation all day long.

Smoking and diabetes are a deadly combination for the vascular system. If you have diabetes and smoke you are greatly increasing the risk of amputation! Fortunately, there are many new medications and good programs to help people quit smoking. If you smoke and you're ready to quit, ask your health care provider to refer you to one of these programs.

Preventing PVD is much easier than treating it. That is why your health care provider will stress that you quit smoking, keep your blood pressure and blood glucose on target, control your cholesterol and triglycerides, lose weight, and stay active. Your doctor can prescribe some medications to treat PVD. Taking an aspirin a day can help prevent heart attacks and strokes, so some people think that it might help prevent PVD, too. Aspirin is not recommended for everyone and can interact with other medications you may be taking, so ask your provider before you start taking aspirin daily.

If you have intermittent claudication (pain in your calves with walking), you might be asked to walk even more. Usually you are encouraged to walk to the point of pain, pause, and then walk a little more. Ask your provider to give you instructions. Walking may help stimulate new vessels to grow and this will improve circulation.

If the tests for PVD show that you have blockage in the larger arteries to your feet or legs, surgeons may try to correct it. One surgery cleans out the artery that is blocked. Another method—angioplasty—involves passing a deflated balloon on a tube to the point where the blockage occurs. The balloon is carefully inflated to open the narrowed artery, and sometimes a stent (a tiny metal device shaped like a spring) is inserted in the artery to keep it open. This surgery is most successful with a small blockage in a healthy artery. A third surgical method is to bypass the blocked area by using a blood vessel from another part of the body (or an artificial blood vessel). While complicated, this surgery can help save a foot, a leg, or a life. People with diabetes often have blockages in the arteries of the lower legs and feet, making it difficult to restore circulation. The relatively new ability to do bypass surgery on the small arteries of the foot has saved many legs. Not all vascular surgeons do this surgery, so check to be sure that yours can. Your providers will carefully evaluate your condition before recommending surgery.

Deformities

A foot deformity is any change in the normal shape of the foot. For people with diabetes, a deformity may be complicated by the additional risk factors of poor sensation and poor circulation. It is the combination of these factors that can make foot deformities dangerous.

Common deformities include bunions, hammertoes, claw toes or mallet toes, curving of the toes toward each other, tailor's bunions, enlargements or bumps of bone behind the heels or on the top or bottom of the foot, and Charcot deformities, which may look like a collapsing of the foot at the arch. These deformities are associated with increased pressure and sheer stress on the skin, resulting in skin breakdown.

A bunion is a deformity in the joint of the big toe that causes the toe to point away from the arch instead of straight ahead. There is usually an unsightly bump on the inside of the foot, just behind the big toe. It is believed that uneven weight distribution during walking and stresses in the joints cause bunions. Heredity is an issue in the cause of bunions, so if you have a family member who suffers with bunions, your risk of developing them is higher. Wearing shoes with pointed toes probably contributes to developing bunions. Tight shoes can exacerbate bunion pain.

If you have a painful bunion or it is difficult to get your shoes to fit, discuss what to do with your foot doctor. Don't put it off. You may need special shoes, orthotics, or padding. Deformities like bunions are a major risk factor for ulcers and amputation. Early corrective surgery may be advised for people with diabetes. Modern bunion surgery not only removes the bump but also attempts to correct the mechanical problem that caused it so that the bunion does not grow back. Severe bunions that have been there for years may even require joint replacement surgery, similar to replacing an arthritic knee joint. Bunion surgery can take about 6 to 8 weeks to heal, so you will want to have your blood glucose levels as close to normal as possible before and after the surgery to encourage healing. You may also have an enlargement behind the little toe. These are called bunionettes or tailor's bunions. They are treated in the same way as regular bunions.

Other common foot deformities include hammertoes, mallet toes, and claw toes. Hammertoes are a bending of a toe at the knuckle closest to the foot. A mallet toe bends at the knuckle closest to the end of the toe and a claw toe bends at both knuckles. As the toe presses up against the inside of the shoe a corn may form over the prominent joint. Pressure from the corn may cause pain or, if the area is numb due to neuropathy, the area may ulcerate. Because the bone is so close to the skin the bone can become infected (osteomyelitis).

Corns between the toes that touch each other are called soft corns or kissing corns. Bones in adjacent toes rubbing together cause these corns, also called heloma molles. Shoes that squeeze the toes together aggravate soft corns. Sometimes they are very painful. The skin may ulcerate and cause infections.

For all toe deformities you can change shoes, add padding, or have surgery. Switch to shoes that have a soft and high rounded toe box that does not press on your toes. You can buy special toe pads made of silicone or soft foam rubber, or you can loosely lace some lamb's wool between or on top of the toes to decrease the rubbing. Do not use cotton or tissues between the toes because these materials can pack down and actually increase the pressure. Inspect your feet every day, including between the toes. See your podiatrist or another health care provider if you think the corn needs to be trimmed, or if it is irritated or ulcerated.

Surgery to correct the problem causing the corn is often the best solution to prevent the corn from occurring. Elective foot surgery is often more important for people with diabetes than for the general population. Many foot ulcers begin as a callus or corn, so preventing the corn can prevent ulcers, infections, and amputations.

Foot deformities, such as hammertoes, can be caused by motor neuropathy. Motor neuropathy affects the way the muscles work. The muscles actually atrophy. Patients with longstanding diabetes and motor neuropathy may lose as much as half of the muscle volume of their feet. When the muscles of the foot do not work properly, an imbalance occurs and toes are often pulled out of their normal position, causing hammertoes. When the toes move upward, they also pull with them soft tissue structures like the fat pad on the ball of the foot. This increases pressure on the bottom of the foot, and calluses and ulcers often form. These are deformities that must be addressed.

If you have calluses try to decrease the high pressure on that spot by wearing shoes with a soft insole and a cushioned outer sole. Don't wear house shoes with little cushioning or go barefoot, because this will make the callus worse. A hard callus is like having a pebble in your shoe. Most foot ulcers occur in the damaged tissue beneath a callus. You need to be evaluated by a foot care professional to see what is causing the callus.

To deal with a callus, you can change shoes, purchase orthotics, moisturize the skin, have a professional trim the callus, or have surgery. Moisturizing the callused area with a good lotion will help keep it soft. Never try to remove a callus by cutting or trimming it with a razor blade. See your podiatrist or health care provider for ongoing callus care. Always avoid over-the-counter corn and callus cures. These products contain acids that can damage the skin. Bathroom surgery may be hazardous to your health! Go to a professional for your foot care.

A serious deformity often associated with diabetic neuropathy is a Charcot's joint or Charcot foot. This is the term used to describe a severe deformity in a weight-bearing joint. A French physician named J. M. Charcot first described the condition in 1868, and later described it involving the foot in 1883. Charcot foot refers to the breakdown of the arch and normal foot structure in a person with nerve damage. Because Charcot's joint usually happens to people who have nerve damage, there is not much pain, even though they may have broken bones and dislocated joints. There is redness, swelling, and increased warmth of the foot. Your shoes won't fit. That's when people usually go to see their provider.

Stay off that foot. The breakdown may occur fairly quickly. Sometimes it is difficult to tell the difference between Charcot's joint and infection. Your foot specialist may order special tests, such as x-rays, MRIs, or bone scans, to make a definitive diagnosis. A bone biopsy of the foot may also be ordered.

Treatments for Charcot's joint are to immobilize the foot in a cast or special boot and rest the foot so it can heal. Sometimes surgery is done to realign the joints of the foot. You may also be prescribed medication to increase bone density and speed up healing. If you continue to walk on a foot with Charcot's joint, you will make it much worse. If you can't get your regular shoes on, or if you have any changes in foot shape or redness, swelling, or warmth, contact your health care provider immediately.

Discuss the options for treatment of any deformity with your foot specialist. If you have adequate circulation, surgery may be your best bet to fix the deformity. Alternatives to surgery include: off the shelf or custom-made special pads or cushions, shoes with extra depth and specially fabricated innersoles, or even custom-made shoes or braces. Prevention of deformities is always preferable to treating them after they are already a problem.

Foot Ulcers

A foot ulcer is an open sore somewhere on your foot. The term "ulcer" refers to a wound or hole in the skin. We often hear about a stomach ulcer, which is a hole in the lining of the stomach. A foot ulcer is a break in the skin that is usually, but not always, shaped like a crater. Foot ulcers often occur in high-pressure areas, so it is common to find one under a callus or surrounded by callus. The most common foot ulcer locations are on the bottom or side of the big toe and on the ball of the foot, especially under the big toe joint. The ball of the foot under the little toe joint is also a common place for foot ulcers. If you have a hammertoe, shoe pressure can rub and cause an ulcer. Diabetic foot ulcers can occur anywhere on the feet. Be aware that the actual break in the skin can be very small, but a larger ulcer may be hidden from view under the surrounding callus or skin. This is why it is important to have your feet inspected by a professional if you think you might have a foot ulcer.

Diabetic foot ulcers are the most common precursor of amputation. 85% of amputations are preceded by an active foot ulcer. Up to 10% of people with diabetes will have an amputation at some time in their lives. Toe and partial foot amputations are the most common. Treatment of ulcers is of vital importance. The lifetime risk of a person with diabetes developing a foot ulcer may be as high as 25%. The most common triad of causes that interact and ultimately result in ulceration includes neuropathy, deformity, and trauma.

If you develop a foot ulcer, the first step in treating it is to cleanse the area gently with soap and water. Apply a clean gauze dressing and avoid pressure to the area. Have the ulcer examined by a health care professional immediately. Once you have received treatment, the wound should begin to show signs of healing in a week or two. Complete healing, however, may take more time. You must follow the treatment plan exactly as prescribed by your foot specialist. Usually, the doctor will trim or cut away the dead tissue, apply a dressing, and, if the wound is infected, prescribe antibiotics. X-rays or an MRI may be ordered. It is important to know if the ulcer has caused an infection in the bone. There are many dressing materials that may help heal your wound. You will likely be asked to change your shoes. You must not walk on an ulcer without protection. The doctor may even apply a cast or a strap-on cast walker to the affected foot and leg. Use bed rest, crutches, or a wheelchair, but stay off that foot.

If the wound has not improved after a few weeks, your doctor will change the treatment plan. There are many new wound treatments that promote healing. Artificial skin products may be used to cover the hole while it heals. Extra oxygen to the wound, either pumped into a boot at home or applied under pressure in a hyperbaric oxygen chamber, can stimulate healing. A vascular surgeon may need to evaluate the ulcer to determine whether surgery might restore circulation to the foot and help heal the ulcer. You may also need a nutritional consultation to make sure your intake of protein, vitamins, and minerals is adequate for optimal healing. Vitamin D, vitamin C, B vitamins, and zinc are believed to be important for wound healing. If a bony protrusion is causing the ulcer, surgery may be needed to change the position of the bone or remove it. Although surgery is not pleasant, it can be necessary to save a limb. Be sure that you are doing all you can to follow the plan and help your foot to heal.

Once the ulcer has healed it is important to keep it closed. Having a history of foot ulcers is the greatest risk factor for getting another ulcer. About 70% of people who have a healed ulcer get another ulcer within

5 years. Since an ulcer precedes most amputations, prevention is very important.

Your podiatrist will want to see you frequently to monitor your foot health. If the cause of the original ulcer is known, it should be corrected if possible, even if it involves bone surgery. Pressure relief is very important, and you will probably need special insoles or shoes to protect your feet. They should be worn all the time; people who wear the shoes consistently decrease their chances of the ulcer reopening. Many insurance companies, including Medicare, will help pay for these shoes and inserts.

Inspect your feet at least once a day. If necessary, use a mirror to see the bottom of your feet or have a family member help you. If you notice any changes, such as a break in the skin or increased redness or warmth, notify your doctor at once.

Infection

People with diabetes who consistently have high blood glucose levels are more likely to develop infections than people with normal blood glucose levels. High blood glucose can interfere with your body's natural defense systems, making infections harder to heal.

Healthy skin is your main defense against infection, and diabetes can make your skin dry and more susceptible to cracking. Germs can enter through small cracks in the skin. Fungal diseases that appear in folds of skin and on your feet need glucose and moisture to grow, and they like high blood glucose levels. The damage they do to your skin can allow an infection to begin.

Common signs of infection are:

- Redness

- Swelling

- Increased warmth

- Pain, tenderness, or limited motion of the affected part

- Foul odor

- Pus or drainage from the wound

If you have one or two of these signs, have your health care provider check your wound as soon as possible to determine whether you have an infection. Other signs that an infection has spread beyond the wound are fever, chills, or unusually high blood glucose levels. If you have any of these signs or symptoms, you should be seen by your health care provider right away. If they are unable to see you immediately, go at once to an emergency room.

New medications and treatments are constantly becoming available. Until recently, bacteria that were resistant to many antibiotics had to be treated by long-term intravenous medications. Now there are oral antibiotics that work just as well, or better, than these intravenous drugs to treat diabetic foot infections and infections caused by resistant germs. Bacteria can develop resistance to new medications as well, so they must be used wisely.

Diabetic foot infections may also be treated by the application of oxygen, either topically or under pressure (hyperbaric oxygen). Some foot surgeons mix antibiotics into a kind of bead that is placed in an infected wound to kill the bacteria directly. Silver also kills bacteria and many wound dressings now contain silver. In addition, open wounds may benefit from the application of negative pressure wound therapy (NPWT). NPWT involves the application of a foam pad to the wound and a plastic wrap over the pad to form an airtight seal. A plastic tube runs from the foam to a small device that applies air suction. This pulls excessive fluid and pus from the wound, pulls skin edges together, and promotes the formation of good healing tissue.

Keeping up with new technologies is a never-ending learning process. Of course, doctors who treat infections and wounds don't rely solely on new therapies. Tried-and-true wound treatments are still the basis for healing most infections. These include removing damaged tissue from the wound, flushing of the wound, off-loading the foot, and the use of topical antiseptics and antibiotics.

Fungus is another type of infection. Abundant worldwide, most fungi are inconspicuous because of the small size of their structures. Since fungi can be found on many of the surfaces you walk on, you can catch the infection simply by going barefoot. You may not even know you have been infected for some time. The only way to tell for sure is to have your health care provider examine you. However, itchy, burning, red, soggy, flaky, or cracking skin or dry scales between your toes are most likely athlete's foot fungus. Because athlete's foot is so common, many providers will treat these symptoms without actually testing for it. Athlete's foot can also occur on the soles or sides of the feet with many of the same symptoms and problems. Often what looks like dry skin is really a fungal infection.

If you think you have a fungal infection you can buy over-the-counter antifungal powders, sprays, and creams. Do not use harsh chemicals like chlorine bleach. Bleach does not kill the fungus and can burn your skin. Apply only a thin layer of medicine. When athlete's foot flares up, apply the medication at least twice a day (morning and night) for at least 4 weeks.

See your provider if you have redness, swelling, or a warm area anywhere on your foot, or if you see any pus. If you have fever or chills or your blood glucose levels are higher than usual, you may have an infection that needs to be treated. Your provider can prescribe stronger antifungal creams and pills for severe cases of athlete's foot. Unfortunately, it may come back when treatment stops.

Some people find that lacing a little lamb's wool between the toes helps keep that area dry. Don't use cotton balls or tissues because they stay moist and can pack down and increase pressure between the toes. Once you have treated the fungus on your feet, you may need to disinfect your shoes and socks or buy new ones. If your toenails are infected, these must be treated also or they will act as a reservoir for the fungus and the skin will become infected again.

There are several things you can do to prevent athlete's foot fungus from becoming a problem. The main one is to keep your feet clean and dry. Wear socks made of fibers that wick the moisture away from your skin. (Cotton stays moist and will keep your skin moist). Put on a clean pair of socks every day. If your feet get wet during the day, change socks more often. There are now socks with a copper or silver weave that kills bacteria and fungi in the sock. Fungi thrive in dark, moist, and warm areas. Wear shoes with leather or fabric uppers that allow air to pass through. Allow your shoes to dry between wearings. If you have two pair, alternate between them. Avoid walking barefoot, especially in public areas such as pools, showers, and locker rooms. Even walking around your own house without protection may allow you to come in contact with fungi brought in on shoes from outside. Fungal infections are contagious. If you don't come in contact with the fungus, you won't catch it.

Fungal infections of the skin and nails may also be the cause of foot odor. Bacteria on the skin also contribute to foot odor. Daily bathing, changing socks, and keeping the feet clean and dry can control this. Using soap and a soft brush to gently scrub away dead skin may help.

If foot odor continues, you might try an antiperspirant for feet or a foot powder designed to control foot odor. Special insoles with activated charcoal or silver and socks that are designed to help control foot odor are available. Foot odor is sometimes a symptom of a serious problem such as a foot infection or foot ulcer that has gone undetected because of nerve damage. Inspect your feet carefully and see your provider immediately if you detect a foot wound.

If you walk without shoes you may also get a plantar wart on the bottom of the foot. Plantar warts are caused by the papilloma virus, which gets into the skin. In some people, the warts disappear without any treatment. In others, plantar warts hang around for years even when they are treated. People with diabetes should always seek treatment.

Although there are many home remedies for plantar warts, the best solution is to see your health care provider or podiatrist. If left alone, a wart may spread into multiple warts that cover large areas of the foot. Warts are caused by a virus, meaning they are contagious and can be spread to family members. Sometimes it is difficult even for professionals to tell the difference between a plantar wart and a callus. There are several treatments for plantar warts. They can be trimmed, padded, or removed with chemicals, frozen with liquid nitrogen, treated with lasers, or removed by surgery. It is important not to leave a painful scar on the bottom of the foot that can affect walking, so it is best not to try any of these treatments by yourself.

Nail Problems

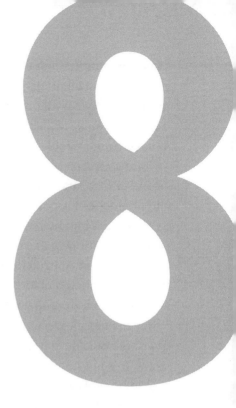

For years, people with diabetes have been told not to cut their own nails. This is not necessarily true. If you have poor circulation, or if your feet are numb from neuropathy, you should not cut your own toenails. Many people have trouble cutting their own toenails safely, especially if they are overweight or have arthritis or vision problems. If you can see and reach your feet well, if you have normal toenails, if you have good nail clippers, and if you are careful, you can trim your own toenails. You could use a large nail file or emery board to file your nails. Filing is less risky than cutting. Nail files for artificial fingernails are good for toenail filing because they have coarser sandpaper than ordinary emery boards. If you have nerve damage or poor circulation or you can't see or reach your feet, ask for help. Thick deformed toenails often require professional foot care.

You may have a family member or friend who is willing to help and will cut your nails for you. Another choice might be a beauty salon pedicure. Pedicures can be risky. Cuts, scrapes, and bacterial and fungal infections are possible. You may want to bring your own instruments and avoid soaking in the tubs at these salons.

Ask whether your provider has a nurse or assistant to trim toenails. In some communities, foot care is available through senior center programs. Almost all podiatrists provide toenail care. Medicare or health insurance may pay all or part of the cost for a podiatrist to trim your toenails if you have diabetes and also meet certain specific criteria, such as having poor circulation.

Trim your nails with the contour of the toe, being sure all sharp edges are cut or filed smooth. The length of the toenail should be even with the end of the toe. It is not a good idea to cut into the edges of the toenail or to try to treat ingrown toenails yourself. This sort of "bathroom surgery" is very risky for people with diabetes. If you injure yourself, seek medical attention for any injury that does not heal promptly. If you have nerve damage or poor circulation and you cut yourself, see your provider right away. Do not wait until you develop an infection.

Try the nail clippers that look like a pair of wire cutters or pliers. They are available in large drugstores, beauty supply houses, and cutlery stores. It is not necessary to have a sterile tool, but your toenail clippers should be kept clean, dry, and sharp. When you use a tool that is dull, you have to put more pressure on the clippers, and can injure yourself if they slip. Do not use pocketknives, kitchen knives, sewing scissors, or pick at your toenails with your fingers. Once you have diabetes, it is too risky to try to cut your toenails with anything except a good pair of toenail clippers.

Do not share clippers with others. Fungal infections of the toenails and skin are contagious and may be passed from person to person.

If you cut yourself while clipping your nails, wash the injury with soap and water and pat it dry. Apply a first aid cream to the wound and apply a bandage to keep it clean, but do not wrap the bandage tightly. Make it loose enough so the circulation is not restricted if the toe or foot swells. Nerve damage may prevent you from feeling pain, however, a wound that does not hurt may still be a serious injury. Change the bandage and inspect the wound every day. Ask for help if you are having trouble seeing or caring for the injury. If you notice any redness, swelling, pus, or an area of increased warmth on your foot, or if the foot does not heal in a reasonable amount of time, report it to your health care provider right away. If you have an infection, you may need to take an oral antibiotic to cure it.

A thick toenail can put lots of pressure on the toe and cause an ulcer, so it is a good idea to have it trimmed down or removed. Whether or not you can trim it yourself depends on how thick it is. Most people need help. It is best to go to a podiatrist or health care provider who is trained to trim thick nails and has special tools to do the job.

A fungal infection usually causes thick toenails. The first step in treating these is to see if a fungus is causing the problem. Your doctor will take a sample of the nail either for microscopic examination or for a culture. Once identified as a fungus, treatment may begin. Creams, oils, and liquid drops are sold over-the-counter to treat fungal toenails. While these may help soften the nail and retard the fungus somewhat, they usually do not make it go away. Your podiatrist or dermatologist may have other suggestions for topical treatments that must be applied daily.

There are prescription pills that may eliminate the fungus on your toenails. Most often these drugs are taken for three months. Because these medications can affect the liver, you will need to have a blood test before you start the medicine and another one about 6 weeks into the 3-month course of treatment. Since toenails grow slowly, the effects of the pills may not be noticed for months. It may take a full year for a nail to grow out normally.

The latest option is a laser treatment. Offered by some podiatrists and dermatologists the laser is passed over the nail. The light penetrates to kill the fungus in the nail and soft tissues around it. This treatment is painless, with no side effects, but you will still need to wait for up to a year for a new nail to grow out to see the full effects. Insurance companies have not been paying for the laser treatment of nails, so this will be an out of pocket expense to you.

Be aware that the fungus might return after any of these treatments. You should talk to your doctor about what you can do to minimize the possibility of the fungus coming back. This may include continuing topical medications, powders to keep feet dry, and the sterilizing of shoes. You may use either sprays made especially to fumigate shoes or ultraviolet lights that are placed in the shoes to kill the fungus in your shoes. In severe or recurrent cases, your doctor may suggest removing the nail and the root of the nail to prevent regrowth.

Ingrown toenails are a common problem for people who have diabetes. This painful condition occurs when the nail grows into the skin. You're more likely to get an ingrown toenail if you trim the toenails too short and cut down the sides of the toenail. Trim your toenails a bit longer, following the curve of the toe without leaving any sharp corners. If the toenail grows into the skin, it breaks the skin, and infection may develop. If the nail has simply been cut incorrectly, a podiatrist or other health care provider can remove the ingrown portion. If you have nerve damage, the ingrown toenail may not hurt, but it certainly needs professional care.

If the problem comes back, the podiatrist will numb the toe and remove a corner of the nail. Sometimes a chemical is put into the corner to kill the root of the nail, called the matrix, and keep the ingrown portion from coming back. Fixing the problem permanently will not only prevent future pain but also may eliminate the possibility of infection. This is especially important for people with diabetes.

After a toenail injury, it is not uncommon for the nail to fall off. Sometimes this happens with very thick fungal nails. Toenails grow slowly—much more slowly than fingernails. It will usually grow back within 12–18 months. Keep the area clean and dry while waiting for the new nail to grow back. Protect it from any further damage by not going barefoot and by wearing shoes that have plenty of room for your toes. The nail-growing cells at the matrix may have been damaged during the injury, so sometimes the new toenail will be a different shape. Remember, if you have circulation problems, any foot injury should be checked by your foot specialist or your primary care provider. If they are not available seriously consider a visit to the emergency room or an urgent care center.

Shoes and Socks

The shoes you choose to wear are of vital importance to your foot health, as well as your general well being, especially if you're a person with diabetes.

The best shoes to wear when you have diabetes are a lace-up shoe with a high, rounded toe box. The upper part of the shoe should be a soft, breathable material such as leather or fabric instead of plastic or synthetic materials. Avoid sandals, clogs, thongs, or flip-flops, because they do not provide the same protection that a closed shoe does. If you have a callus or deformity, you need a shoe with a soft innersole that redistributes the pressure on the sole of your foot. With a bunion or hammertoe, you may need extra-width or extra-depth shoes, or a shoe with a stretch material, such as Lycra, for the toe area.

If you have trouble tying laces, try shoes with Velcro fasteners. Most tied shoes can be converted to Velcro fasteners at a shoe repair shop. Elastic shoelaces allow you to get your shoes off and on without untying the laces.

Avoid tight, pointed shoes. High heels are not good for any foot. They force the entire weight of the body onto the front of the foot, changing the shape, greatly increasing pressure, and causing ulcers. Look for a shoe that is shaped like a foot. While this sounds reasonable, it can be a challenging task, especially for women. Your podiatrist or a pedorthist (certified shoe fitter) can help you pick the right shoe. It's worth the effort. Good-quality athletic shoes or walking shoes are often excellent choices as well.

People with diabetes should wear shoes all the time. Even carpeting at home does not prevent you from stepping on pins, tacks, toys, dog bones, and whatever the cat brought in. Doctors often remove small pieces of glass, wood splinters, and even needles from dropped insulin syringes from the feet of people who have walked without shoes at home. Over 80% of amputations can be traced back to a minor traumatic event!

Also, most people do not take their shoes off before they enter their homes. The shoes track in viruses, fungi, and bacteria, which are deposited on floor surfaces. Viruses can cause warts, fungi can cause athlete's foot and nail diseases, and bacteria can cause infections. If you walk barefoot in your home, you may come in contact with these disease-producing organisms.

Make it a habit to protect your feet at all times—at the beach or pool (water shoes), in public showers (shower shoes), and even in your own home (house shoes or slippers). The only time to go without shoes is when you are in bed or bathing.

Of course, proper shoe fit is also important. Have both feet measured every time you buy shoes, and shop for shoes in the afternoon or evening when your feet may be swollen. Your shoes need to fit all day. Wear the socks that you will be using with the shoes you are buying. When you try on shoes, check that the ball of the foot rests in the widest part of the shoe. Walk a few steps and look for signs of a poor fit, such as the foot rolling over the sole or too much space between the heel and the back of the shoe. Notice whether the shoe bends where your foot does, and be sure there is plenty of room for your toes. There should be a half-inch space between the longest toe and the end of the toe box, but the shoes should not slip. (The longest toe is not always the big toe.) Be sure the toe box is high enough and does not press on your toes.

If you have foot deformities, or have had an ulcer that is now healed, you should have shoes prescribed and fitted or custom-made by a podiatrist, orthopedic surgeon, or pedorthist. If you have nerve damage, even your properly fitted new shoes may feel too big. Also remember that people's feet tend to get longer, wider, and flatter as the years go by. You will not always wear the same size.

Most people with diabetes do not need custom-made shoes. Custom-made shoes are necessary only for people with significant deformities that cannot be accommodated by a stock shoe. However, if you are at risk for ulceration or amputation, you may need special, therapeutic shoes—for example, ones with extra depth and inserts. You are considered to be at risk if you have already had a toe or partial-foot amputation, if you have a foot deformity, if you have ever had an ulcer that is now healed, or if you have diabetes-related foot problems such as poor circulation (peripheral vascular disease) or nerve damage (diabetic neuropathy). A podiatrist or other health care provider who can examine your feet is the best person to advise you about custom shoes.

Prescription footwear can help prevent some foot problems. Medicare pays for therapeutic footwear when you meet certain criteria and have your diabetes care provider complete the proper forms. This benefit covers custom-molded shoes, extra-depth shoes, inserts, and some shoe modifications. Your physician must certify on the form that you are in a diabetes care plan, have evidence of foot disease, and need therapeutic footwear. Only a doctor who is treating you for diabetes can make this certification. The doctor must also have in his records the reason(s) that you qualify for the shoes/inserts. You can get the certification form from prescription shoe stores, Medicare, your podiatrist, or the physician treating your diabetes. Often, the podiatrist or pedorthist will help you get the forms completed by your diabetes care provider.

A podiatrist then writes the prescription for the therapeutic shoes, and a podiatrist or pedorthist supplies them. You must buy the footwear from a qualified supplier. Some suppliers require you to pay for the shoes and inserts and then get reimbursed by Medicare; others will wait for Medicare to pay them directly, so that you do not have to pay the money upfront. In either case, Medicare covers 80% of the allowed amount, while you or your secondary insurance, if you have one, must pay the balance. Suppliers who participate in Medicare cannot charge more than Medicare allows. Suppliers who do not accept Medicare assignment may charge more than Medicare allows, and you must pay the difference.

You may also need insoles for your shoes. You can relieve pressure on the soles of your feet by wearing a cushioning layer between your foot and the floor. If you wear thin-soled shoes, or if you have high-pressure areas on your feet, it is a good idea to add insoles to your shoes. High-pressure areas are where calluses develop. Most ulcers begin under a callus. If you can prevent or reduce the size of a callus, you may prevent an ulcer from developing in that area, too.

Some insoles are available in drugstores, grocery stores, sporting goods stores, and running shoe stores for less than $10 a pair. Running shoe stores also have insoles with extra arch support for $15 to $30. Some stores now "scan" your feet and offer "suggestions" for which of their insoles to buy. Be sure to check with your foot care specialist before buying any insole. Your podiatrist may have specific recommendations and some insurance companies pay for special innersoles for people with diabetes. An insole will raise your foot in the shoe, so be sure that you have plenty of room in the toe of the shoes. If your shoes are too tight with the insoles, you would do better with half-insoles that do not go under the toes. Many insole materials lose their cushioning effect and will need replacement every 3 to 4 months. If you have foot deformities, a foot imbalance, pressure areas or calluses on your feet, you may need orthotics.

Orthotics are specially designed insoles that are worn inside your shoes to control the way your foot moves or to support painful or at-risk areas of the foot. Often mistakenly equated with non-custom arch supports, they can do much more than cushion and support. Additions, top covers, extensions, or wedges can be added to the orthotics to hold your feet in a more stable position inside the shoe. This can help you walk normally, relieve foot pain, avoid calluses and corns, and even help with knee, hip, and lower back pain.

Orthotics are usually custom-made using a plaster model, a foam impression, or a computer scan of your feet. They may be made of a rigid material, like plastic, but can also be made of leather or other soft materials. Graphite orthotics are durable and can be made very thin for comfort and improved shoe fit. Properly made orthotics should be comfortable. Orthotics should always be prescribed by a foot care specialist. Never buy these devices through the mail or from stores without a prescription.

Check to see whether your health plan will help you pay for orthotics. Often they will be covered. One pair may not fit inside all your shoes, so you may want separate orthotics for dress shoes or sports. Orthotics must be replaced periodically, so ask the person who made them when you'll need new ones. Orthotics change the way your feet and lower extremities work, so it's best to break them in gradually. Wear them for only an hour the first day, and increase your time on them by an hour each day until you are wearing them all day.

What should you do if your feet are different sizes? It is very common for one foot to be slightly larger or wider than the other. Small differences can easily be accommodated by the podiatrist or pedorthist. If you need two different-sized shoes or if you have only one foot, you might want to contact the National Odd Shoe Exchange (www.oddshoe.org) or the One Shoe Crew (sally_tvarez@hotmail.com). These organizations help their members with mismatched or odd-sized feet to find shoes. Some members are matched with another member who has exactly the opposite shoe size problem so that they can share shoe purchases rather than having to buy two different-sized pairs to come up with one wearable pair. These groups are also of value to people with amputations who may need only one shoe. Nordstrom's Department Stores also sells mixed size pairs of shoes.

Another alternative is a custom made pair of shoes. These shoes can be especially helpful for people with severe deformities who cannot wear regular off-the-shelf shoes. Those with partial foot amputations may find custom shoes beneficial. These shoes are made from casts or molds of the feet.

Be careful about jumping on the bandwagon and purchasing shoes that are the latest fad. Among these fads are the "minimalist" or barefoot walking shoes and the "exercise" or "shape up" shoes. Both of these shoe types have been reported to cause injuries. Stick to shoes recommended by your foot doctor.

You should inspect your shoes every day. Look for anything that might injure your feet, especially if you have lost feeling in them. Look over the top and sole of the shoe, shake it out, and run your hand into it. Look and feel for any pebbles, or other foreign objects, and check for nails or tacks in the sole of the shoe. Look for cracked uppers or rough seams that could rub a blister. Replace shoes with worn or loose linings. If heels or soles are worn down, get new shoes or have them resoled so that your foot gets the support it needs. If your podiatrist has prescribed special insoles or orthotics, periodically pull these out and check them as well. The soft inserts that often come with therapeutic shoes flatten out and must be replaced three times a year. If you meet the qualifications for therapeutic shoes outlined above Medicare will pay 80% of the cost of three pairs of these insoles every calendar year. If you have a secondary insurance plan they may pick up the other 20%.

Choose your socks wisely. Socks should be made from acrylic or synthetic material that wicks moisture away from your skin; cotton just holds the moisture on the skin. Some manufacturers are now making socks with a silver or copper fiber woven into the material. These fibers kill fungi and bacteria, keeping feet healthier and reducing odor.

Socks should not be too tight or too loose and should fit without folds or wrinkles. Choose socks without seams. Garters or socks that bind may cut off circulation to your feet and legs. If the elastic at the top of your socks is too tight, cut a notch into the cuff of the sock.

Socks shaped like feet are preferable to tube socks, which tend to thin out over the heel and bunch up in the front. Change into clean socks daily. Throw away socks with holes. Do not wear socks that have been repaired. Repaired socks may have rough patches that can irritate your foot.

Sock color is generally irrelevant. Some people, however, are allergic to the dye in some socks and, therefore, only wear white socks. If you do not have an allergy to the dye, you may wear any color you choose. Some people with diabetic neuropathy and insensitive feet also choose to wear white socks. Wearing white helps them see blood or drainage on their socks if they get a cut or a sore on their feet. Daily foot exams, which are recommended for everyone with diabetes, should eliminate the need to depend on sock stains to tell if there is a foot wound.

You can find extra large socks in big and tall shops, athletic stores, and department stores. Sports stores may have socks that are double knit on the bottom to provide an extra layer of cushioning. Drugstores also carry diabetic socks at the pharmacy. Just be sure that they don't make your shoes too tight. When you are purchasing new shoes, try them on with socks of the thickness that you will be wearing.

Wear nylon stockings or panty hose for the shortest time possible. Nylon is not a breathable fabric (that's why they make raincoats out of it!), so change into some socks as soon as you can.

Additional Risk Factors

As mentioned in other chapters in this book the people who are most at risk for foot problems have diabetic nerve damage. If poor circulation is also present, the danger increases. Compound the problem by adding in foot deformities and the risk is greatest. Other risk factors include limited joint mobility, thick nails, a history of having a foot ulcer or amputation, or having other complications of diabetes, such as eye disease (retinopathy) or kidney disease (nephropathy).

Once you have had a foot ulcer or amputation, you are likely to get another one. This is because you have serious damage to the nerves and blood vessels of your feet, or the mechanics and shape of your foot have changed, not because you do not take care of your feet. Most people with diabetes who have had foot problems take better than average care of their feet, but good foot care alone may not be enough to prevent foot problems once they are already established.

The changes in your biomechanics (the way your foot works) or shape of your foot following amputation should be clear to almost everyone. If a toe, for example, is amputated the rest of the foot clearly will not function as it did previously. As pressure points change stress is placed on new areas and they may become callused or develop blisters or sores.

For this reason, ulcers are much more common in people who have had amputations.

Newly diagnosed young people with type 1 diabetes who do not have other complications of diabetes or other foot problems have low risk. The American Diabetes Association recommends that annual foot risk screening begin 5 years after the diagnosis of diabetes, but it is never too early to develop good foot care habits.

Older people who are recently diagnosed with type 2 diabetes may actually have had diabetes for years before finding out about it and may already have complications. If you have type 2 diabetes, start good foot care right away.

Do you believe that excessive weight affects your feet? Absolutely. This is just common sense, and not just for people with diabetes. The more we weigh, the more stress is transmitted through our knees, ankles, and feet. Many people with foot pain can get relief just by losing weight. Heel pain is one example of a pain that is often weight related. Arthritis pain in the knees and feet is frequently worse in people who are overweight.

People who are obese have a different gait from those who are not. Their feet are placed wider than normal because their thighs hold the legs outward. This places the body weight more toward the inner part of the foot, changing the mechanics of walking completely. There is increased stress on the tendons, ligaments, and joints of the feet. Custom foot orthotics can help improve the mechanics of gait.

If you have diabetic neuropathy, your weight is even more important. The stress of additional pounds on numb feet increases the likelihood of your developing ulcers and Charcot deformities. Even losing a small percentage of your body weight can make a huge difference in foot pressure and may decrease the possibility of ulcers and amputation.

If you become pregnant, your feet may change shape and size during the pregnancy and for about 6 months after the baby is born. Sometimes they remain permanently larger. Why? During pregnancy, your body retains fluid, and your feet swell. Most often this swelling reverses after delivery. Also, the hormone relaxin, which is needed to soften and stretch the pubis aiding in delivery, also loosens the joints in your feet which may spread out—sometimes permanently. Be aware of this and try to wear comfortable, supportive shoes, such as running shoes. High heels are not really a good idea for anyone, but especially not for a pregnant woman.

Since the size of your feet may have changed, it is even more important to have your feet measured when buying shoes after childbirth.

Can your job also contribute to foot problems? Sure. Do you work in an environment where your feet get wet a lot? Moisture and dark places, like the inside of a shoe or work boot, can breed fungi. Freezing temperatures can lead to cold-related injuries such as frostbite. Trauma from falling objects on the job can cause injuries such as fractures and lacerations. Even the foot gear that you wear should be carefully evaluated and fit to make sure there is no pressure from items such as protective steel toes. This is especially important if you have numbness from neuropathy.

Changes can occur in our hardworking feet as we age, especially joint diseases like arthritis. Bones can shift out of position, rubbing against shoes and causing pain and the buildup of calluses or corns. We lose some of the fat pad that cushions the ball and heel of the foot—and people with diabetes may lose it all—causing a callus to grow as a way to relieve the sharp pressure of bones on the soles of our feet. This and other changes can make us unsteady, and our gait or walking pattern may change. Our feet tend to get longer, wider, and flatter, which affects how our shoes fit.

You can offset some of the effects of aging. Always wear shoes that fit well; have your feet measured every time you buy shoes. Sometimes changes in the shape of your feet occur so gradually that you do not notice how poorly your shoes fit, especially if you have nerve damage and cannot feel your feet. Don't wear shoes that you have saved for years for special occasions.

An unsteady gait can be a sign of another type of medical problem, so talk to your provider about it. Falls can lead to fractures and even death. It may just be time to get a cane or walker. Numb feet due to neuropathy may be the reason your gait is unsteady. Your provider or physical therapist can give you tips on getting a cane of proper length and how to walk with it. If you believe you are unsteady, or if friends or family members tell you that you are, ask your provider about a referral to a physical therapist for balance training.

One of the best ways to keep your muscles, bones, and joints young is to stay active. This is also good for your diabetes. If you have never been active, you can begin by exercising sitting down. Yoga or Tai Chi are excellent activities that can be done even by the elderly.

Your diet may also affect your feet. You know that achieving near-normal blood glucose levels can improve your chances of not having nerve damage or circulation problems. Part of managing your blood glucose is following a meal plan, along with exercising daily and taking diabetes medication if you need it.

What you eat affects your health, including your skin, muscles, and bones. A meal plan that is unbalanced, with too many processed foods (white flour, sugars, and fats) and too few vegetables and fruits, leaves you with fewer weapons to use against bacteria and fungus on the skin. Healthy eating for people with diabetes means eating the same healthy foods that everyone should eat. Especially important are the vitamins and the minerals that you can get from vegetables and fruits. You also want to be sure that you are getting enough calcium and magnesium to keep your bones strong. Ask for a referral to a registered dietitian (RD) if you need help designing or changing your meal plan to meet your needs and to manage your blood glucose levels. What you eat also affects your blood fats and plays an important part in circulation and peripheral vascular disease.

A discussion of risk factors would be incomplete without talking about smoking. In fact the use of tobacco, in any form, may be impli-cated in many amputations. Smoking is clearly connected to develop-ing vascular (heart and blood vessel) disease. When you smoke, the combustion products of tobacco are absorbed into the bloodstream. These chemicals stimulate the release of other chemicals, which injure the blood vessels and encourage thickening and hardening of the arter-ies. Smoking also causes your blood vessels to constrict or clamp down, limiting the amount of blood that can circulate. Smoking even as few as two cigarettes a day can constrict the blood vessels all day long. This constriction cuts off vital blood supply and can stop wounds from heal-ing, leading to gangrene.

Smoking and diabetes are a deadly combination for the vascular sys-tem. If you have diabetes and smoke you are greatly increasing the risk of amputation! Fortunately, there are many new medications and good programs to help people quit smoking. If you smoke and you're ready to quit, ask your health care provider to refer you to one of these programs to help you do it.

Skin care

Most of us do not think of skin as an organ, but it is. In fact it is our largest organ, weighing in at about 8 pounds. It doesn't rest internally, but surrounds our insides to make us waterproof, guard against infection, chemicals and sunlight, manufacture vitamin D, and help us look pretty good.

There are three layers to the skin. The outermost layer, or epidermis, is made of the protein keratin, which is also what makes up nails and hair. The next layer down is the dermis where we find sweat glands and hair follicles. The deepest layer, the subcutis, has fat that cushions and protects.

The skin is clearly vital to your well-being. As a person with diabetes, having healthy skin is even more important. People with diabetes who have high blood glucose levels most of the time are more likely to develop infections than people with normal blood glucose levels. High blood glucose can interfere with your body's natural defense systems so that infections are harder to heal.

Healthy skin is your main defense against infection, and diabetes can make your skin dry and more susceptible to cracking. Once the skin is broken, germs can enter. Fungal diseases that appear in folds of skin and on your feet need glucose and moisture to grow, and they like high blood glucose levels. The damage they do to your skin can allow an infection to begin.

As we age, skin may become thinner and dryer, so your dry skin may be from normal aging. People tend to have more dry skin in winter because of heating systems blowing dry air. Bathing with very hot water or soaking can also contribute to dry skin because it washes away natural skin oils. Harsh soaps and detergents also remove these oils.

People with diabetes can develop a type of nerve damage called autonomic neuropathy. The autonomic nerves control blood flow, sweating, and skin moisture. People who have autonomic neuropathy may notice that their feet sweat less or not at all. This can cause severe dry skin.

Remember that fungal infections (athlete's foot) may look like simple dry skin (see the chapter on infections). One common type of fungus, *Tricophyton rubrum*, typically has what is described as a "moccasin" appearance. That means that the distribution looks like a slipper or moccasin. The dryness, scales, or flakes are on the bottom and sides of the foot but may not cover the top. If you are not sure if it is dry skin or a fungus ask your health care provider.

Moisturize dry skin daily to prevent itching and cracking and to help keep germs out. Moisturizers are packaged as creams, lotions, ointments, and oils. For most people, any good body or hand lotion will do, as long as you remember to use it. Select a kind that you like and will actually use every day.

Avoid lotion with alcohol because it evaporates and takes moisture from the skin. Some people are sensitive to chemicals in highly perfumed or colored lotions, but there are lotions with no smell or color. Avoid lotions with lanolin if you are allergic to wool. Lotions with mineral oil may not work as well as lotions containing olive oil, almond oil, jojoba oil, or vegetable oils. Aloe vera gel is another good moisturizer.

The best time to apply lotion is after a bath or a shower, to help seal in the moisture your body has absorbed. Do not apply moisturizers between your toes; these areas usually need no help in staying moist. Apply lotion one to three times a day. Keeping lotion in your sock drawer may help you remember to use it. If you prefer to apply lotion at bedtime, put on a pair of socks to keep the lotion off the sheets and help it soak in overnight.

Ask your health care provider or pharmacist to recommend a moisturizer. Products that contain lactic acid or urea help moisturize better than those with just emollients. You can get a prescription moisturizer if you have special problems or severe dry skin. Your health care provider or pharmacist may be able to help check your insurance plan to see if there are moisturizers that they will help pay for.

Good foot hygiene, keeping your feet clean, is important. The best way to wash your feet is in the bathtub or shower. Wash your feet just like you wash the rest of your body. If your feet have lost sensation due to neuropathy you may not be able to tell if the water is too hot. Check the temperature with your elbow. The elderly and the obese may have trouble getting to their feet. Family members or caregivers may be able to help. There are also devices that can help you reach your feet, such as a long handled brush or sponge. Other types of brushes have suction cups that hold the brush down while you rub your feet against them. Check with an occupational therapist or a medical supply company for suggestions regarding assistive devices.

If you have dry skin, you might want to try soap with moisturizer to combat dryness. Soap that is not milled is more moisturizing. Milling removes glycerin to make the soap harder and easier to shape. Antibacterial soaps are not necessary. If you have a fungal infection (athletes' foot) there are soaps that have anti-fungal properties that may be of benefit along with the medications prescribed by your provider.

You can also wash your feet in a pan of water. Take the same precautions and be sure that the water is not too hot. If you cannot use the bathtub or shower, any plastic or metal tub the size of a dishpan will work. Don't soak your feet. This can dry out the skin excessively and even lead to infections. Be sure to rinse your feet well, and be sure to dry very well, especially between the toes. Use a soft fluffy towel to gently pat your feet dry. Don't rub. Moisturize after washing.

Some people experience an increase in perspiration. This may be a sign that your blood glucose levels are not on target, sometimes occurring when blood glucose levels are too low (hypoglycemia). Most of the time, diabetic nerve disease decreases foot sweating. Obesity, infectious diseases, hormonal changes associated with menopause, and increased thyroid function can cause increased perspiration. If you have sweaty feet, wear shoes made of leather or fabric that "breathes." Avoid shoes made of plastic or synthetic materials. Try to change your shoes during the day. If that is not possible, rotate between two pairs of shoes, wearing one pair every other day. (Keeping your feet dry helps prevent fungal infections, but you should avoid excessively dry skin that may crack.)

Wear socks that wick the moisture away from your skin. If you have athlete's foot, or want to try to prevent it, look for socks with silver or copper fibers. These materials kill fungi and bacteria in the sock. Change socks frequently: at least daily and maybe two or three times a day, if necessary. If you have to wear nylon stockings, change into socks as soon as you can.

You may have to use an antiperspirant. Try a regular underarm antiperspirant first. If that doesn't work, you may need a prescription antiperspirant. Follow the directions on the package and stop using the product immediately if you experience any skin irritation. Severe hyperhidrosis can be treated with Botox injections, which help for 6–7 months.

Friction on your skin may cause a blister. If you develop a blister and have neuropathy or poor circulation, see your health care provider right away! Don't wait until it gets infected. Stop wearing the offending shoe immediately. Wash the area with warm water and mild soap and dry well. Do not break the blister—this can allow germs to get under the skin. Cover the blister with a dry bandage. If the blister breaks, leave the loose skin as a covering over the wound until it heals. It is not necessary to apply antiseptics, antibiotic ointments, or chemicals to the blister.

Inspect the blistered area daily. If there is redness, tenderness, swelling, pus, or a warm area around the wound after the first day, you may be getting an infection. See your provider for evaluation. Over-the-counter antibiotic creams are not strong enough to treat a foot infection in a person with diabetes. If the wound is deep, gets larger, or does not heal within a few days, have it checked without delay.

Don't wear the offending shoes again until the blister is entirely healed. You might need extra padding, different socks, or something else to keep them from rubbing. Wear the shoes for a short while; then check your feet for signs of another blister. It is better to throw them away than to continue wearing shoes that injure your feet.

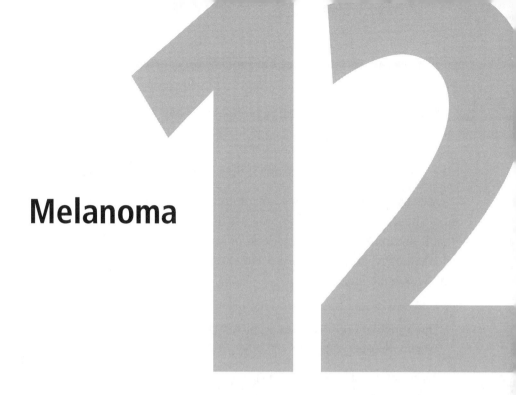

Melanoma

Skin cancer is often caused by too much exposure to ultraviolet (UV) rays from the sun or tanning beds. This exposure can include intense UV radiation obtained during short periods, or lower amounts of radiation obtained over longer periods. According to the American College of Foot and Ankle Surgeons, "Melanoma is a cancer that begins in the cells of the skin that produce pigmentation (coloration)." If the cancer continues to grow beneath the surface of the skin and spread to other areas of the body, it is malignant melanoma. Unlike many other types of cancer, melanoma strikes people of all age groups, even the young.

Melanoma that occurs in the foot or ankle often goes unnoticed during its earliest stage, when it may be more easily treated. By the time melanoma of the foot or ankle is diagnosed, it frequently has progressed to an advanced stage, accounting for a higher mortality rate. This makes it extremely important to follow prevention and early detection measures involving the feet, as well as other parts of the body.

Anyone can get melanoma, but some factors put a person at greater risk for developing this type of cancer. These include:

> Fair skin; skin that freckles; blond or red hair

> Blistering sunburns before the age of 18

> Numerous moles, especially if they appeared at a young age

Melanoma can occur anywhere on the skin, even in areas of the body not exposed to the sun. Melanoma usually looks like a spot on the skin that is predominantly brown, black, or blue—although in some cases it can be mostly red or even white. However, not all areas of discoloration on the skin are melanoma.

There are four signs—known as the ABCDs of melanoma—to look for when self-inspecting moles and other spots on the body:

Asymmetry—Melanoma is usually asymmetric, which means one half is different in shape from the other half.

Border—Border irregularity often indicates melanoma. The border (or edge) is typically ragged, notched, or blurred.

Color—Melanoma is typically a mix of colors or hues, rather than a single, solid color.

Diameter—Melanoma grows in diameter, whereas moles remain small. A spot that is larger than 5 millimeters (the size of a pencil eraser) is cause for concern.

If any of these signs are present on the foot, it is important to see a foot and ankle surgeon right away. It is also essential to see a surgeon if there is discoloration of any size underneath a toenail (unless the discoloration was caused by trauma, such as stubbing a toe or having something fall on it).

To diagnose melanoma, the foot and ankle surgeon will ask the patient a few questions. For example: Is the spot old or new? Have you noticed any changes in size or color? If so, how rapidly has this change occurred?

The surgeon will also examine the spot to determine whether a biopsy is necessary. If a biopsy is performed and it reveals melanoma, the surgeon will discuss a treatment plan. Remember: Early detection is crucial with malignant melanoma. If you see any of the ABCD signs—or if you have discoloration beneath a toenail that is unrelated to trauma—be sure to visit a foot and ankle surgeon as soon as possible. An alternative would be to visit a dermatologist for evaluation.

The Aging Foot

Changes can occur in our hardworking feet as we age, especially joint diseases like arthritis. There are dozens of types of arthritis. Arthritis may wreak havoc on your feet. Bones can shift out of position, rubbing against shoes and causing pain and the buildup of calluses or corns. These deformities are a major risk factor for amputations in people with diabetes.

As we age, we lose some of the fat pad that cushions the ball of the foot—and people with diabetes may lose it all—causing a callus to grow as a way to relieve the sharp pressure of bones on the soles of our feet. This and other changes can make you unsteady and may have an effect on your walking pattern. Our feet tend to get longer, wider, and flatter, which affects how our shoes fit.

Most people have a decrease in circulation in their legs and feet as they age. This is especially true for people with diabetes. See the chapter on circulation problems to learn more about this important topic.

It is possible to offset some of the effects of aging. Always wear shoes that fit well. Changes in the shape of your feet often occur so gradually that you do not notice how poorly your shoes fit, especially if you have nerve damage and cannot feel your feet.

An unsteady gait can be a sign of another type of medical problem; perhaps you have diabetic neuropathy affecting the ability to feel your feet as you walk. It may just be time to get a cane. Your provider or physical therapist can give you tips on getting a cane of proper length and can teach you how to walk with it.

We all want to live to our full potential. Falls threaten the independence and even the lives of older adults. How big is the problem? According to the CDC:

> Among those age 65 and older, falls are the leading cause of injury death. They are also the most common cause of nonfatal injuries and hospital admissions for trauma.

> One out of three adults age 65 and older falls each year.

> In 2007, over 18,000 older adults died from unintentional fall injuries.

> The death rates from falls among older men and women have risen sharply over the past decade.

> In 2009, 2.2 million nonfatal fall injuries among older adults were treated in emergency departments and more than 581,000 of these patients were hospitalized.

> In 2000, direct medical costs of falls totaled a little over $19 billion—$179 million for fatal falls and $19 billion for nonfatal fall injuries.

Many falls are preventable. The CDC says: "Older adults can take several steps to protect their independence and reduce their chances of falling. They can:

> Exercise regularly. It's important that the exercises focus on increasing leg strength and improving balance. Tai Chi programs are especially good.

> Ask their doctor or pharmacist to review their medicines—both prescription and over-the counter—to reduce side effects and interactions that may cause dizziness or drowsiness.

▶ Have their eyes checked by an eye doctor at least once a year and update their eyeglasses to maximize their vision.

▶ Make their homes safer by reducing tripping hazards, adding grab bars and railings, and improving the lighting in their homes."

Make sure your podiatrist has you in the right shoes, insoles, or even braces for stability. Remember that many insurance companies, including Medicare, pay for shoes for people with diabetes that qualify.

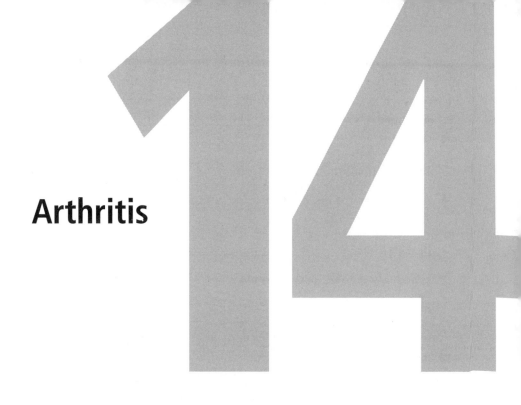

Arthritis

"Arthro" refers to joints, "-itis" means inflammation. Arthritis is an inflammation of a joint. This is usually characterized by swelling, pain, and restriction of motion. There are over 100 different kinds of arthritis and different treatments for each kind. It is best to let your health care provider diagnose and treat any problems you are having with your joints. Don't assume that any pain, swelling, or stiffness in your foot is "just arthritis." There are many over-the-counter medications for treating arthritis, but consult your health care provider if you take these regularly.

Since both arthritis and diabetes tend to affect people as they age, it is common to have both conditions. Arthritis can make it difficult for people with diabetes to stay as active as they need to be. However, because exercising and staying active are treatments for both arthritis and diabetes, you get a double dose of benefits whenever you exercise.

There are many new medications for arthritis. The current thinking is that arthritis should be treated more aggressively than it was in years past. Researchers think that starting treatment early could prevent much of the pain and disability associated with arthritis.

According to the National Institutes For Health (http://www.ncbi. nlm.nih.gov/pubmedhealth/PMH0002223/), "arthritis involves the breakdown of cartilage." Cartilage normally protects a joint, allowing it to move smoothly. Cartilage also absorbs shock when pressure is placed on the joint, such as when you walk. Without the normal amount of cartilage, the bones rub together, causing pain, swelling (inflammation), and stiffness.

"Joint inflammation may result from:

➤ An autoimmune disease (the body's immune system mistakenly attacks healthy tissue)

➤ Broken bone

➤ General 'wear and tear' on joints

➤ Infection, usually by bacteria or virus

Joint inflammation typically goes away after the cause goes away or is treated. When it doesn't, it becomes chronic arthritis. Arthritis may occur in men or women. Osteoarthritis is the most common type."

Other, common types of arthritis include:

➤ Rheumatoid arthritis

➤ Gout

➤ Psoriatic arthritis

➤ Arthritis caused by infection

➤ Neurogenic arthritis

In addition to the joint pain, redness, swelling, and decreased motion of the joint there may also be a deformity of the joint. Since foot deformities are one of the major risk factors for ulceration, infection, and amputation, arthritis with deformities must be taken very seriously. Charcot deformity is a type of arthritis (see the chapter on deformities for more information on Charcot deformities).

An accurate diagnosis of arthritis is important so that treatment may be directed appropriately. Your doctor will do a thorough examination and may order x-rays, blood tests, MRI's, or CT scans and may send a sample of your joint fluid to a lab for testing.

Gout is a special type of arthritis caused by an excess of uric acid in the blood. Uric acid crystals tend to settle in joints; the big toe or bunion joint is the most common site. These crystals can cause the big toe joint to become extremely painful, red, warm, and swollen. If you have the symptoms of gout, your health care provider will likely x-ray the area. Gout has special signs on x-ray that the doctor will look for. She or he may withdraw some joint fluid and examine it under a microscope to look for these crystals. Medications and a special diet to lower the uric acid levels in the body are the main treatments for gout. Avoiding foods such as animal proteins (especially organ meats), seafood, and alcohol (especially beer) can help prevent attacks.

Sometimes it is difficult to tell the difference between gout and an infection caused by bacteria. If you think you might have gout, it is important to see your health care provider. Repeated episodes of gout tend to damage the big toe joint and may make it stiff. This can cause a high-pressure spot on your foot that is more prone to developing a callus and an ulcer. Be sure to check your feet daily for any signs of redness or ulceration. If the joint does become stiff, you may need surgery to help loosen it or to replace it with an artificial joint.

With any type of arthritis pain relief is a primary goal. In addition your health care provider will, if possible, address the cause and prevent or decrease the severity of flare ups.

According to the NIH "lifestyle changes are the preferred treatment for osteoarthritis and other types of joint inflammation. Exercise can help relieve stiffness, reduce pain and fatigue, and improve muscle and bone strength. Your health care team can help you design an exercise program that is best for you."

Exercise programs may include:

> Low-impact aerobic activity (also called endurance exercise)

> Range of motion exercises for flexibility

> Strength training for muscle tone

Physical therapy may be recommended. This might include:

> Heat or ice

> Splints or orthotics to support joints and help improve their position; this is often needed for rheumatoid arthritis

- Water therapy
- Massage

Other recommendations:

- Get plenty of sleep. Sleeping 8 to 10 hours a night and taking naps during the day can help you recover from a flare-up more quickly and may even help prevent flare ups.

- Avoid staying in one position for too long.

- Avoid positions or movements that place extra stress on your sore joints.

- Modify your home to make activities easier. For example, install grab bars in the shower, the tub, and near the toilet.

- Try stress-reducing activities, such as meditation, yoga, or tai chi.

- Eat a healthy diet full of fruits and vegetables, which contain important vitamins and minerals, especially vitamin E.

- Eat foods rich in omega-3 fatty acids, such as coldwater fish (salmon, mackerel, and herring), flaxseed, rapeseed (canola) oil, soybeans, soybean oil, pumpkin seeds, and walnuts.

- Apply capsaicin cream over your painful joints. You may feel improvement after applying the cream for 3-7 days.

- Lose weight, if you are overweight. Weight loss can greatly improve joint pain in the legs and feet."

Your podiatrist should also suggest appropriate shoes and inserts or orthotics to accommodate any deformities and to remove pressure from bony prominences. There are also many accommodative pads, now available in cushiony gel materials, which may also be used for protection and comfort. Definitive treatment, however, may involve surgery (see the chapter on surgery that follows).

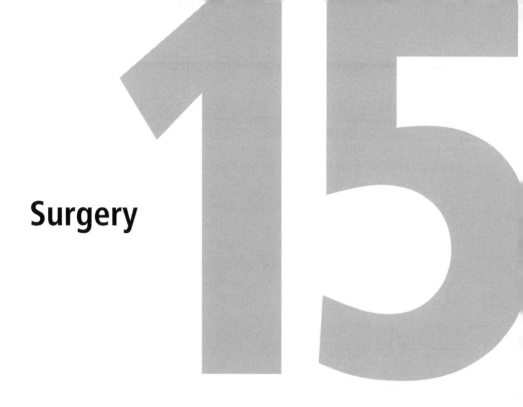

Surgery

Surgical correction of foot deformities is often your best defense against ulceration, infection, and amputation. A hammertoe, for example, may rub against a neighboring toe or against the inside of the shoe, forming a corn or callus. These hard layers of skin precede most ulcers. The pressure forms an ulcer that, in turn, may become infected and require amputation. If surgery is performed before the ulcer and infection can occur, the toe, foot, or leg may be saved. Any surgery entails some risk; however, the risk of not having a deformity corrected is also high. Non-surgical care often does not address the true problem and may be only temporary in nature.

Preventive surgery for people with diabetes is now widely accepted. Most deformities worsen over time, as do the effects of neuropathy and vascular or circulatory disease, so early surgery before these complications progress is often best.

Surgery is indicated for pain relief, for pressure relief, to allow for appropriate shoe gear, to remove bone or soft tissue infections, and for amputations in the case of gangrene.

People with diabetes often develop problems that are unrelated to their diabetes but may still require surgery. Painful hammertoes or bunions, ingrown toenails, skin cancer, or trauma are examples of such problems.

Modern foot surgery is often performed on an outpatient basis. A hammertoe may be corrected by a small stab incision, about 1/8 inch long, allowing a contracted tendon to be cut. Almost no down time is needed for this. If a small piece of bone needs to be removed, the time off will increase. Bunion surgery requires more work and, generally, more time off. The bone must be cut, moved, and held in place with pins or screws.

Surgery for ingrown toenails requires no down time at all. Removing the ingrown portion of the nail is a common procedure. The toe is numbed and the procedure is often performed right in the doctor's office. Normal activities may be resumed immediately.

While many foot surgeries are simple procedures, there are many other really complicated procedures. A Charcot deformity, for example, can require a complex reconstruction, with the insertion of screws, pins, and plates to hold the bones together during healing. An external fixation device may be needed. This reconstructive procedure certainly involves more disability.

Adequate circulation is necessary when healing from any surgery. Because people with diabetes often develop circulation problems sooner than the general population, your doctor may recommend that you have foot surgery sooner rather than later. Before surgery, your foot surgeon should explain nonsurgical options, evaluate your circulation, discuss your diabetes management with you, and explain the postoperative care you will need to follow. If you have any doubts about the suggested surgery, get a second opinion from another qualified foot specialist.

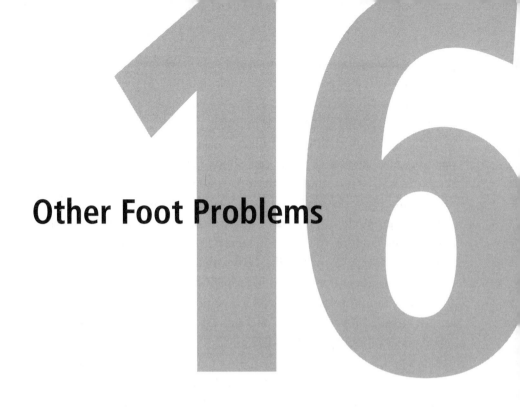

Other Foot Problems

People with diabetes have heard the stories about hospitalizations, extended disabilities, and amputations. Foot problems may not be a complication of diabetes at all. After all, many people who do not have diabetes visit podiatry offices and emergency rooms with foot complaints and injuries. Sometimes it is hard to differentiate between a problem directly caused by diabetes and one that is not.

Foot pain and/or numbness in patients with diabetes are often diagnosed as diabetic peripheral neuropathy. There are many types of neuropathy (www.neuropathy.org), and determining the cause of the problem may require the expertise of a neurologist or physiatrist. Numbness may occur in an isolated area of the foot, perhaps only in two toes. These neurological symptoms are associated with an ailment called a neuroma.

Also known as a "Morton's Neuroma," this is a disorder that often affects the nerve that supplies sensation to the 3rd and 4th toes. This nerve becomes thicker and causes numbness and pain. Although we do not know exactly what causes neuroma formation, it is more common in women as well as those with abnormally flat or high arches and is associated with tight shoes and high heels.

One sign of a neuroma is a "Mulder's click." A doctor will squeeze your foot and push on the nerve on the bottom of the foot. The nerve may slide and "pop" between the metatarsal bones. Some people can even feel this click as they walk. A diagnostic ultrasound or MRI may be helpful. X-rays will not show a neuroma.

Treating a neuroma may include a change in shoe type, orthotics, padding, or injections of either cortisone or alcohol. The latter destroys the nerve so that it cannot transmit pain sensations. Surgical removal of the neuroma may be necessary.

In addition to neuromas, other nerve disorders may mimic diabetic neuropathy. Trauma, vitamin deficiencies, alcoholism, autoimmune diseases, and toxic chemicals like heavy metals or chemotherapy drugs used to treat cancer may lead to neuropathic symptoms. Compression of a nerve, often in the back, can lead to symptoms of neuropathy. This is known as radiculopathy. Another compression of the nerves to the feet is called tarsal tunnel syndrome (TTS).

Most people have heard of carpal tunnel syndrome, a nerve compression at the wrist, but are unaware that a similar compression may occur at the tarsal tunnel in the ankle. TTS occurs when the tibial nerve is compressed as it passes through the area behind the inner ankle bone, or medial malleolus. Pain, numbness, and tingling in the foot can occur with TTS. (Sounds like diabetic neuropathy, doesn't it?) People may feel electric shock sensations or a "pins and needles" feeling. This electric shock sensation or a tingling along the nerve can sometimes be duplicated by tapping on the nerve. This is called a Tinel's Sign.

Testing for TTS may include nerve conduction studies. These studies time the transmission of impulses along the nerve. If the transmission is delayed, the study is abnormal. It is important to make sure that the problem is at the ankle region and not higher up, even in the back. The nerve conduction tests will tell your doctor where the problem lies along the nerve. Treatment includes the use of orthotics, rest, pain medications, and various physical therapy modalities. If these conservative treatments are unsuccessful, surgery to release the nerve may be necessary.

There are over 100 types of arthritis. Arthritis may mimic some of the problems people with diabetes encounter with their feet. Pain, stiffness, and deformities are common effects of arthritis. Arthritis has several different treatments depending on the type, so an accurate diagnosis it very important. Making sure the problem is not a complication of diabetes, such as a Charcot joint, is especially important. X-rays along with more sophisticated tests like bone scans and MRIs are often used to differentiate one type of arthritis from another.

If you have diabetes, and stub a toe and it becomes deformed because of a dislocation or fracture, you may not remember the seemingly minor injury and assume the problem is related to your diabetes. While a foot injury may put someone with diabetes at risk for major problems, the injury itself may not have been the result of a diabetes complication. The same is true for skin irritations and blisters.

Some insect bites have consequences that can be quite severe. Spider bites inflict injuries that may resemble a diabetic type of wound. The incidence in the U.S. is unknown. Symptoms may range from mild pain around the bite, swelling, burning, itching, redness, and tenderness to ulceration of the skin, infection, and swollen lymph glands in the groin (assuming the bite was on the lower extremity). Two types of spiders found in the U.S. that may cause severe bites are the Black Widow and the Brown Recluse. The bite of the Brown Recluse may cause an ulceration that can take months to heal and may require skin grafting.

Some types of skin cancer may also look like wounds we see in people with diabetes. Certainly, if you have diabetes, ANY sore should be evaluated by a doctor. It is often difficult, even for professionals, to differentiate between types of lesions. What may look like a simple birthmark can be a deadly melanoma. What looks like a diabetic ulcer can be malignant. Many doctors will biopsy an ulcer that has not healed to see if there has been malignant transformation of the wound.

The list of foot problems that can masquerade as diabetes-related disorders can be extensive. Almost any foot problem that people without diabetes get can fool a person with diabetes into believing it is their diabetes that is causing it. Foot care professionals will be able to accurately diagnose the problem and devise a treatment strategy to keep you on your feet.

Over-the-Counter Products

Walk down the aisles of your supermarket, pharmacy, or large mart stores and you will undoubtedly run into the large displays of foot care products.

Foot care products have always been big business. "Several factors have converged to drive this growth. Consumer interest in private-label products; a large Baby Boomer population with associated aches and pains of aging; clinical product innovations to serve the needs of diabetics and alternately, spa-like product innovations to serve consumers interested in pampering their feet will continue to push the market forward.... The market may reach even greater heights if the players step up their advertising and promotional budgets (http://packagedfacts.com/Footcare-products-1432869/)." This is big business.

Everyone with diabetes should use their podiatrist as a resource. Your foot doctor will know which products are safe and effective. Your doctor may be able to supply or prescribe a superior product or device that is also covered by your health insurance. For example, many insurers will pay for shoes and shoe inserts for people with diabetes.

An orthotic, or orthosis, is a device or support for the foot that is specifically designed to relieve or correct an orthopedic problem. Although over-the-counter inserts may be less expensive, orthotics prescribed by your doctor are made from a mold of your feet and will be custom manufactured to your doctor's prescription.

Many over-the-products contain a product label that states, "Not for use by people with diabetes." Corn and callus removers, corn plasters, wart removers, and similar products contain harsh chemicals, usually acids. They decrease the buildup of hard skin by softening and burning away the corn or callus. If you have diabetic nerve damage, you might not be able to feel it if the chemical has burned too much or spread to the surrounding normal skin. It is dangerous for a person with diabetes to get any breaks in the skin because of the risks of infection and difficulty with healing.

Whenever possible, you should treat the cause of the problem so that corns and calluses do not form. These products just try to remove the hard skin. See your podiatrist if you have a corn or callus that needs to be treated. Remember that ulcers, infections, and amputations are often preceded by calluses, so get them treated professionally.

Although not generally dangerous, anti-fungal nail products sold over-the-counter have very low success rates. Your doctor may be able to prescribe an effective product that also will be covered by your prescription drug plan, so you end up paying less for a better result.

If your feet perspire, or have an odor, you may try an antiperspirant. Try a regular underarm antiperspirant first. If that doesn't work, you may need a prescription antiperspirant. Follow the directions on the package and stop using the product immediately if you experience any skin irritation.

If the problem continues, try an antiperspirant for feet or a foot powder designed to control foot odor. Special insoles with activated charcoal, silver, or copper, and socks that incorporate these materials help control foot odor. Wear socks that wick the moisture away from your skin (special acrylic blends or CoolMax). Change socks frequently; at least daily and maybe two or three times a day if necessary. If you have to wear nylon stockings, change into socks as soon as you can.

Then there is the supplement market, advertised to promote either a healthy lifestyle or directed at a specific problem. Who hasn't heard and seen the ads for products to keep your bones strong, or your joints healthy, or your cholesterol at that right level to prevent heart disease?

Research has shown that some supplements are helpful, while others have no effect or can even harm your health. Beware the hype and check with your health care provider before taking ANY OTC product. Some supplements may have adverse effects upon your current medications, increasing or decreasing their effectiveness.

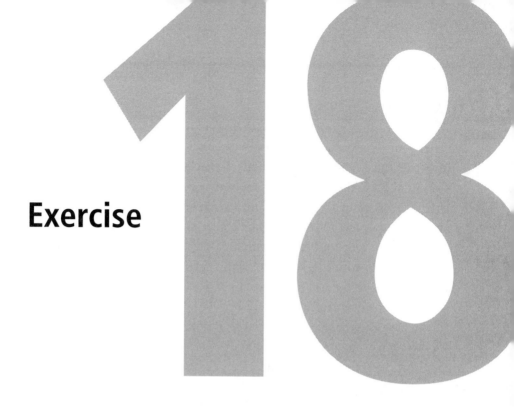

Exercise

What are the best ways to control your blood glucose levels? Take your medications and stick to your diet and exercise. You also know that exercise will help you look and feel better too.

One of the best ways to keep your muscles, bones, and joints young is to stay active. This is also good for your diabetes. If you have never been active, you can begin by exercising sitting down. Weight-bearing exercise, however, also improves your bone strength. If you should take a tumble, good bone strength may prevent fractures. Research has proven that exercise will prevent the changes in muscles and bone that we see with aging.

When it comes to exercise, it's best to start slowly. Walking is free and you can do it anywhere. Find a friend to exercise with. You will both motivate each other. Many communities and shopping malls have walking clubs. Get some light weights or exercise bands for resistance training that you can do at home. Are you able to join a gym? The trainers there can help you get started. There is no age limit on these suggestions. Studies have shown that people in their 80's and 90's can benefit from an exercise program. Tai Chi has been especially recommended for older people. The sooner you start the better. Start off slowly and build up as you get stronger. You'll be glad you did!

You may need to follow some foot precautions before you start a walking or running program. Have a thorough foot exam to discover any deformity, lack of feeling, or poor circulation. Wear socks with good cushioning that are made from a material such as acrylic or CoolMax. Good-quality walking or running shoes may prevent injury. Always take the time to warm up. Cool down and stretch after the exercise activity and inspect your feet for redness, blisters, or hot spots. If you have pain during exercise, stop and try to figure out what is wrong. You may need orthotics to help your feet work normally during physical activity—especially if you are active and have knee pain or pain in the arch or heel area of your foot (plantar fasciitis).

If you have a loss of feeling in your feet, limit repetitive weight-bearing exercises such as jogging and using stair-climbers because of the high pressure on your feet and possible injury that you wouldn't be able to feel. Do not do weight-bearing exercises when you have a foot ulcer. When the ulcer has healed, make sure to ask your doctor what caused it and take special precautions when exercising to keep it from coming back. People with a history of ulcers are more prone to getting one again.

Walking can actually improve circulation in your legs and feet by forcing the blood vessels to work harder and expand. In fact, this is the recommended exercise for people with intermittent claudication (pain in the calf due to poor circulation). Walking is good for your heart and for your diabetes management as well. Try to walk for 30 to 60 minutes every day. If you don't have an hour to spare at one time, try two 15- to 20-minute walks.

If you have lost much of the feeling in your feet, you can participate in non-weight-bearing exercises, such as swimming, bicycling, or rowing; upper-body exercises, such as weight lifting; and range of motion and stretching exercises, such as yoga or Tai-Chi. You will achieve your best level of fitness if you do several different types of exercise during the week. For example, you can do stretching exercises one day and strength-building exercises the next day. Aerobic exercise (e.g., walking, running, biking, or swimming) should be performed every day (Yes, every day). In a pool, you should wear aqua shoes to protect your feet.

Remember that your household chores, such as vacuuming and gardening, count as exercise as well.

You should always wear good-quality athletic shoes that are made for the activity you are doing. This means wearing running shoes for running, golfing shoes for golfing, and bowling shoes for bowling. Almost every sport is associated with a special type of shoe appropriate to the particular activity. These shoes are important for preventing injury. And they may help you perform better and enjoy the sport more!

A good running shoe offers support and stability to protect your feet from injury. For many people with diabetes this may be their best bet for an everyday shoe choice. Be sure to buy your shoes from a knowledgeable salesperson at a running store. The fit of the shoe is vital. Leave enough room for your toes. When running downhill the shoe stops and the foot may slide forward and the toe can hit on the inside. Bleeding under the nail, or worse, may indicate the need for a longer shoe.

Remember to examine your feet carefully after each time you exercise. This is especially true if your feet are numb because of diabetic neuropathy.

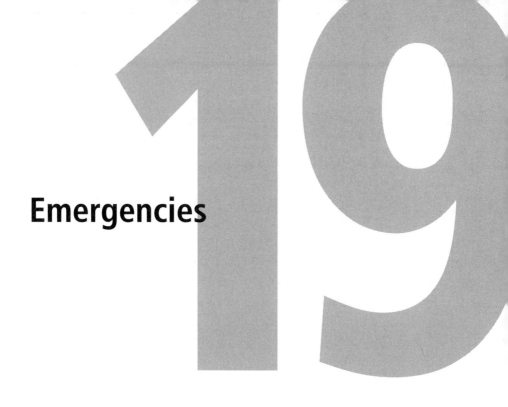

Emergencies

If you have diabetes, a foot related injury can be devastating. This is especially true if you have peripheral vascular disease (PVD), which is poor circulation, or diabetic neuropathy (DN), which is numbness in your feet. You should understand the prevention and treatment of foot trauma.

When should you either call the doctor or go to the emergency room? The answer really depends upon your medical condition before the injury. If you have PVD or DN an injury can be more dangerous to you than to someone who does not have these issues. You should ask your podiatrist or primary medical provider to give you some guidelines for handling potential problems. Ask about various types of emergencies—sprains, cuts, contusions (stubbing a toe), bleeding, blisters, redness, or sudden pain. Some of these can be treated on your own at home, but it's good to know when to treat yourself and when to get to the doctor.

It is important to realize that some minor problems can rapidly progress to really severe, potentially limb threatening, emergencies. Early intervention may prevent disaster later.

People with diabetic nerve damage cannot feel their feet, so they may not notice any pain. They may continue to walk on an injury or high-pressure spot that would cause pain in a person without nerve damage. This continued walking might cause a wound or ulcer. Once the skin is broken, the ulcer can become infected. People with diabetes who have high blood glucose levels most of the time are more likely to develop infections than people with normal blood glucose levels. High blood glucose can interfere with your body's natural defense systems, making infections harder to heal.

This is why some people with diabetic neuropathy wear white socks. Wearing white helps them see blood or drainage on their socks if they get a cut or a sore on their feet. Daily foot exams, which are recommended for everyone with diabetes, should eliminate the need to depend on sock stains to tell if there is a foot wound.

Even minor injuries require care. What should you do if you nick yourself while trimming your toenails? If you have nerve damage or poor circulation, see your health care provider. If you don't, wash the injury with soap and water and pat it dry. It is generally not necessary to apply antiseptic creams to the wound. You may apply a bandage to keep it clean, but do not wrap the bandage too tightly. Make it loose enough so that the circulation is not cut off if the toe or foot swells.

Do not be reassured if the wound does not hurt, because nerve damage may prevent you from feeling it. A wound that does not hurt may still be a serious injury. Change the bandage and inspect the wound every day. Ask for help if you are having trouble seeing or caring for the injury. If you notice any redness, swelling, pus, or an area of increased warmth on your foot, or if the foot does not heal in a reasonable amount of time, report it to your health care provider right away. If you have an infection, you may need to take an antibiotic to cure it.

Despite wearing the right shoes and socks, you may still develop a blister on your foot from time to time. If you have neuropathy or poor circulation, see your health care provider immediately! Don't wait until it gets infected. Wash the area with warm water and mild soap and dry well. Do not break the blister—this can allow germs to get under the skin. Cover the blister with a dry bandage. If the blister breaks, leave the loose skin as a covering over the wound until it heals. It is not necessary to apply antiseptics, antibiotic ointments, or chemicals to the blister.

Inspect the blistered area daily. If there is redness, tenderness, swelling, pus, or a warm area around the wound after the first day, you may be getting an infection. See your provider to get antibiotics. Over-the-counter antibiotic creams are not strong enough to treat a foot infection in a person with diabetes. If the wound is deep, gets larger, or does not heal within a few days, have it checked immediately.

Don't wear the shoes again until the blister is completely healed. You might need extra padding, different socks, or something else to keep them from rubbing. Wear the shoes for a short while; then check your feet for signs of another blister. It is better to throw them away than to continue wearing shoes that injure your feet.

Sometimes people with nerve damage do not feel pain and can injure a foot or toe quite severely without knowing it. If you have nerve damage, check your feet carefully with your eyes and your hands after any injury to see how bad it is. An example of this is a stubbed toe. This injury can be very painful and can vary from minor to severe. If you don't have peripheral vascular disease, put ice on the injury and elevate it higher than your heart to relieve the swelling and pain. Is the toe in an abnormal position? Do you have continued pain, swelling, or an inability to put weight on the foot? If so, you need to see your health care provider for an X-ray of your foot to make sure that you have not broken any bones. If you neglect a fracture, particularly of the big toe, it can result in a painful deformity. You need early treatment to prevent a deformity from occurring.

If blood accumulates under the toenail, it can put pressure on the toe. You may need to visit your health care provider to have the pressure relieved. Do not try to relieve it yourself by puncturing the nail or performing any other home surgery. When you have diabetes, it is best to have a health care provider treat all foot injuries.

After a toenail injury, the nail may fall off. This may happen with very thick fungal nails. Toenails grow slowly—much more slowly than fingernails. It will usually grow back within 12–18 months. Keep the area clean and dry while waiting for the new nail to grow back. Protect it from any further damage by not going barefoot and by wearing shoes that have plenty of room for your toes. The nail-growing cells at the root, or matrix, located at the base of the nail may have been damaged during the injury, so sometimes the new toenail will be a different shape.

If you have a puncture wound from stepping on a foreign body like a nail, see your health care provider right away. Puncture wounds are a serious matter, especially when you have diabetes. Nails and other sharp objects do not have to be rusty to cause lockjaw (tetanus) or to cause an infection in your foot. Punctures through shoes are especially dangerous because a little rubber from the sole of the shoe sometimes enters the wound and causes a nasty infection.

Wash the area with warm water and mild soap and dry well. Cover the wound with a dry bandage. It is not necessary to apply antiseptics or antibiotic ointments. Keep the area covered until you can see your doctor and receive appropriate care and instructions. All adults should have tetanus booster shots repeated at least every 10 years. If you are not sure when you had your last tetanus booster, it is safe to have another one when you are injured.

If you are travelling, you should pack a small foot emergency kit. Many of the items in the kit are appropriate for other minor injuries as well. The kit should include bandages, sterile gauze pads, waterproof tape, alcohol pads, scissors, an antibiotic ointment, 1/4-inch adhesive felt, and a 4-inch ace bandage. When placing tape directly on the skin, paper tape is the best option.

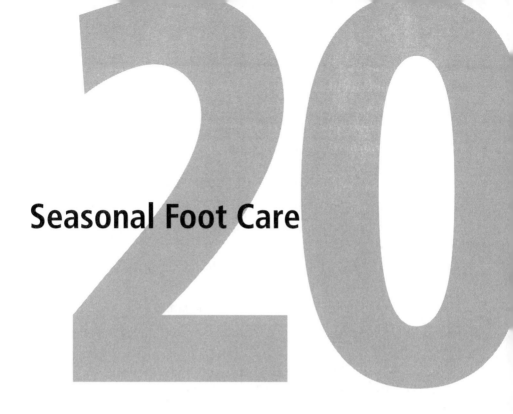

Seasonal Foot Care

With the changing of the seasons, comes the need to alter foot care treatment. From sandals in the summer, to boots in the winter, shoe selection is important, especially for people with diabetes. Do not settle for a flimsy pair of flip flops. These can hurt your feet. There are now many flip flops with arch supports and heel cups that are comfortable and look great too. Your podiatrist can help you choose sandals that offer support and comfort. These will protect your feet, provide better cushioning, improve your balance and decrease the possibility of ankle sprains, and may help with knee and back pain. Better still, talk to your foot specialist about sandals with custom orthotic footbeds.

Even good sandals are not meant for every activity. If you are beginning to return to exercising after a winter at rest, choose appropriate sport specific shoes. Do you have new running shoes? Break them in slowly. Watch out for skin irritations or blisters.

Time off from work and vacations change activity levels for many of us from sedentary winter activities. Summer poses risks to the feet, especially for people with diabetes. Injury is possible to miss, especially if feet are numb because of neuropathy. Foreign bodies, burns, infections from fungi, viruses (warts), and/or bacteria are all possible if you walk without shoes.

Now is the time for those good flip-flops or sandals with arch support and heel cups. Never go barefoot; not even at the beach or pool. Puncture wounds from shells and other debris are especially difficult to treat. Don't forget sunscreen on your feet! Make sure the sunscreen protects against both UVA and UVB rays. Remember to reapply frequently and liberally. Always wear socks when wearing shoes. This will give you an added layer of protection to prevent irritation and wick moisture away form the skin.

The days are now getting shorter. Fall has arrived. You should still be active, if you live in the north, enjoy the changing leaves. But now is also the time to prepare for winter. Get warm shoes and socks ready. Sporting goods stores and ski shops are great sources for winter wear. When purchasing shoes/boots wear the socks you plan to use with them when you try them on…thick socks take extra room. Remember that if you have neuropathy, proper fit is essential…you may not be able to feel if the shoes are too tight. Break in new winter boots gradually and examine your feet frequently. If the boots or shoes are not already waterproof consider adding waterproofing.

Appropriate shoes/boots are a must in winter as well. Avoid getting your feet wet and stay out of the cold as much as possible. Skin tends to be drier in the winter, so apply lotion frequently to avoid dry, cracked skin.

The best thing to do for cold feet is to wear one or two pairs of thick socks or warm house slippers—but check to be sure that your shoes are not too tight. You can try the thin silk socks that are worn under regular socks for added warmth. There are also special socks available that will retain body heat and keep your feet warm. Regular exercise helps keep your feet warmer, too.

Do not use heating pads or hot water bottles on your feet. Don't sit too close to a space heater, fireplace, or campfire. If you have any diabetic nerve damage, you cannot feel when your feet are too hot or are getting burned, and you could be badly injured. In addition to making your feet cold, nerve damage can affect blood flow and sweating in the feet. People with these problems are not able to release heat from their feet by dilating blood vessels the way someone without nerve damage would. It's best to wear socks and move around from time to time.

Cold injury, even frostbite, is possible, especially if feet are numb due to neuropathy. Frostbite can be superficial or deep, which can result in temporary or permanent damage to the skin.

Symptoms of frostbite can include: progressive numbness, tingling or burning sensations, pain which may disappear as the condition progresses, and changes in color of the toes or fingers that may go from red to white or purple. Gangrene can result.

If you suspect frostbite, immediately get indoors. Re-warm the area where the frostbite occurred. Immerse body part in a bath with a constant temperature of 104-105°F for about one hour. Do not use very hot water. Do not smoke because smoking constricts blood vessels and you are trying to dilate them. Be sure to seek medical care as soon as possible.

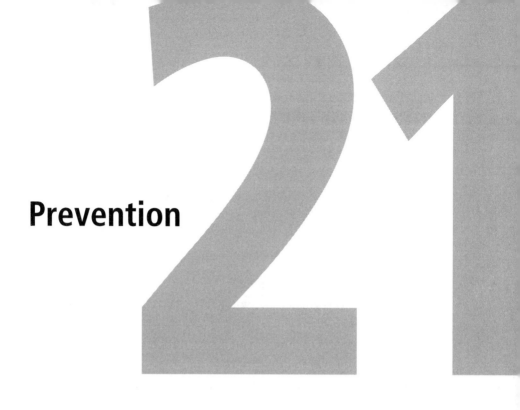

Prevention

Experts believe that at least 50% of amputations in people with diabetes could be prevented by near-normal blood glucose levels, better preventive foot care, and better care of foot ulcers.

You can take several very important steps to protect your feet. Keep your blood glucose levels as close to normal as you can. Inspect your feet every day and after exercising. Get regular medical attention for your feet at least once a year, more often if your doctor has made that suggestion. Many ulcers are preceded by calluses, so be sure you see a podiatrist and treat these calluses aggressively. There is no magic to avoiding foot complications. The key is to develop a routine that includes commonsense, everyday attention to your feet.

Here is a brief checklist of things to do:

➤ Do keep your feet clean and dry.

➤ Do have a complete foot exam at least once a year, more often if you have circulation problems, deformities or numb feet.

➤ Do wear well-fitting shoes and socks.

➤ Don't go barefoot.

- Don't soak your feet.

- Don't use any over-the-counter preparation on your feet without an OK from your podiatrist.

- Don't put lotion between your toes, but put it on the rest of your foot.

- Do get monofilament testing at least once a year.

- Do treat calluses aggressively by seeing a foot care specialist.

- Do get any injury to your foot seen right away!

Remember to examine your feet daily. Look at the tops, bottoms, and between toes. Do this regularly and you will know what "normal" is for you. If you see a change, tell your podiatrist or other care provider so that treatment can begin at once. If you have trouble seeing, have a family member or other caregiver do this exam for you.

Hygiene is very important. Clean feet well daily, but don't soak. This is a good time to do your foot inspection.

Shoes, shoe inserts or orthotics, and socks are crucial to good foot health. Choose these wisely and make sure they are appropriate for you and fit well. You should put new shoes on at home for a while prior to wearing them outside. If they do not feel good after wearing them for an hour or more, or if they cause red spots or irritations, return them.

Regular foot exams are one of the keys to good foot health. It is never too early to develop good foot care habits so as soon as you find out that you have diabetes see a podiatrist for a baseline evaluation. This is especially true for older people who are recently diagnosed with type 2 diabetes and who may actually have had diabetes for years before finding out about it and may already have complications. If you have deformities preventive surgery should be discussed with your foot specialist. If you have peripheral vascular disease you should discuss options with a vascular surgeon.

Periodic podiatric exams should be performed at least once a year… more often if you have neuropathy, circulation problems, or deformities. Your primary care physician and endocrinologist should examine your feet at each visit. To help remind them, take off your shoes before they come in to examine you.

By reading this book you have taken the first step in your education process regarding your foot health; but there is more that you can, and should, do. Learn all you can. For more information, visit the American Diabetes Association online at www.diabetes.org and the American Podiatric Medical Association website at www.apma.org. Both have lots of information about diabetic foot care.

The American Diabetes Association develops and disseminates diabetes care standards, which are published annually. These statements represent the official position of the ADA. The ADA position statement on foot care, "Preventive Foot Care in People with Diabetes," can be found online at http://care.diabetesjournals.org/content/26/suppl_1/s78.full. The foot care statement covers risk identification, foot exams, prevention of high-risk conditions, management of high-risk conditions, patient education, and provider education. Understanding how to prevent problems and what to do about them is crucial for diabetic foot care. This brief statement offers specific recommendations for people with diabetes as well as their care providers. You may want to give a copy of this position statement to all of your care providers.

Never stop controlling your diabetes, exercising, and protecting your feet!

Resources

American Diabetes Association
1701 North Beauregard Street
Alexandria, VA 22311
(800) DIABETES
(703) 549-1500
Website: www.diabetes.org
Bookstore: www.store.diabetes.org

American Academy of Orthopaedic Surgeons
6300 North River Road
Rosemont, IL 60018-4262
(800) 346-AAOS
(847) 823-7186
Website: www.aaos.org

American Association of Diabetes Educators

100 West Monroe, Suite 400
Chicago, IL 60603
(800) 338-3633
Website: www.aadenet.org
E-mail: aade@aadenet.org

American Board of Podiatric Surgery

445 Fillmore Street
San Francisco, CA 94117-3404
(415) 553-7800
Website: www.abps.org
E-mail: info@abps.org

American College of Foot and Ankle Surgeons

8725 West Higgins Road, Suite 555
Chicago, IL 60631
(800) 421-2237
(773) 693-9300
Website: www.acfas.org
E-mail: info@acfas.org

American Orthopaedic Foot and Ankle Society

2517 Eastlake Avenue East, Suite 200
Seattle, WA 98102
(206) 223-1120
(800) 235-4855
Website: www.aofas.org
E-mail: aofas@aofas.org

American Podiatric Medical Association

9312 Old Georgetown Road
Bethesda, MD 20814-1698
(301) 571-9200
(800) FOOTCARE
Website: www.apma.org

Amputee Coalition of America

900 East Hill Avenue, Suite 285
Knoxville, TN 37915-2568
(888) 267-5669
Website: www.amputee-coalition.org

Diabetes Exercise and Sports Association (DESA)

8001 Montcastle Drive
Nashville, TN 37221
(800) 898-4322
Website: www.diabetes-exercise.org
E-mail: desa@diabetes-exercise.org

Lower Extremity Amputation Prevention Program (LEAP)

National Hansen's Disease Programs (NHDP)
1770 Physicians Park Drive
Baton Rouge, LA 70816
(800) 642-2477
Website: bphc.hrsa.gov/leap

National Chronic Pain Outreach Association

P.O. Box 274
Millboro, VA 24460
(540) 862-9437
Website: www.chronicpain.org

National Odd Shoe Exchange

P.O. Box 1120
Chandler, AZ 85244-1120
Website: www.oddshoe.org

Neuropathy Association

60 East 42nd Street, Suite 942
New York, NY 10165
(800) 247-6968 / (212) 692-0662
Website: www.neuropathy.org
E-mail: info@neuropathy.org

One Shoe Crew
  E-mail: Sally_tvarez@hotmail.com

Pedorthic Footwear Association
  7150 Columbia Gateway Drive, Suite G
  Columbia, MD 21046-1151
  (800) 673-8447
  (410) 381-7278
  Website: www.pedorthics.org

President's Council on Physical Fitness and Sports
  200 Independence Avenue, SW
  Room 738-H
  Washington, DC 20201-0004
  (202) 690-9000
  Website: www.fitness.gov

State-Based Diabetes Prevention and Control Programs
  Centers for Disease Control
  CDC Division of Diabetes Translation
  P.O. Box 8728
  Silver Spring, MD 20910
  (877) 232-3422
  Website: www.cdc.gov/diabetes/states/
  E-mail: diabetes@cdc.gov

Take Care of Your Feet for a Lifetime (brochure)
  National Diabetes Education Program
  National Institutes of Health
  Website: www.ndep.nih.gov/diabetes/pubs/Feet_broch_Eng.pdf